American Pharmacy

American Pharmacy
(1852-2002)
A Collection of Historical Essays

Edited by Gregory J. Higby and Elaine C. Stroud

Essays reprinted from the *JAPhA* series commemorating the Sesquicentennial of the American Pharmaceutical Association, with permission.

American Institute of the History of Pharmacy
2005

Publication No. 21 (New Series)
Gregory J. Higby and Elaine C. Stroud, General Editors

American Institute of the History of Pharmacy
777 Highland Ave.
Madison, WI 53705
www.aihp.org

A Fischelis Publication
on Recent History and Trends of Pharmacy

fourth of a series aided by a fund established
in the American Institute of the History of Pharmacy

by

ROBERT P. FISCHELIS (1891-1981)
pharmacist • administrator • author • educator

Table of Contents

Preface   *vii*

CHAPTER 1
Pharmacy Practice   *1*

CHAPTER 2
Pharmaceutical Sciences   *19*

CHAPTER 3
Pharmaceutical Education   *37*

CHAPTER 4
Pharmaceutical Industry   *55*

CHAPTER 5
Governance of Pharmacy   *75*

CHAPTER 6
Pharmacy Organizations   *87*

NAME INDEX   *109*

Preface

THE essays contained in this booklet were first published in the *Journal of the American Pharmaceutical Association* as part of the sesquicentennial celebration of APhA. Working with the editorial staff of the *Journal*, I helped to determine the topics and authors of the series, which was published during 2000, 2001, and 2002. George Griffenhagen contributed valuable input and selected appropriate illustrations from the APhA Foundation Archives.

After receiving requests from instructors, the Institute decided to collate the pieces by topic into a single booklet. Far from a comprehensive text (each general subject deserves its own book-length treatment) this set of essays instead serves as an introduction to six key aspects of pharmacy's history in the United States from 1852 to 2002: Practice, Science, Education, Industry, Organizations, and Governance. Composed by nine different authors, the essays sometimes overlap and repeat information, which reflects the interwoven reality of the complex pharmaceutical enterprise. Rather than edit out these redundancies, we have left them in so that each essay remains useful for teaching and reference purposes. Those readers looking for more comprehensive treatments of these topics are referred to *Kremers and Urdang's History of Pharmacy,* revised by Glenn Sonnedecker, 1976, reprinted 1986 by AIHP and *Pharmacy: An Illustrated History,* by David L. Cowen and William H. Helfand, 1990. For more bibliographic guidance, consult the end of Chapter 2, "Evolution of Pharmacy," in *Remington: The Science and Practice of Pharmacy* or the website of the American Institute of the History of Pharmacy (www.aihp.org).

Special thanks go out the American Pharmacists Association and its Executive Vice President, John A. Gans, for permission to reprint these pieces. Our gratitude is extended as well to the authors for their cooperation. The layout of this booklet was done by Elaine C. Stroud.

Gregory J. Higby
Madison, Wisconsin

Introduction
American Pharmacy Before 1852

*by Gregory J. Higby**

W HEN twenty men gathered in Philadelphia in 1852 to found the APhA, it was a turning point rather than a beginning. These pharmacists took a significant step away from purely commercial concerns toward the goal of achieving professional status for their chosen occupation. It would take decades of progress on several fronts for this goal to be reached. The short essays that follow describe six key areas of this development.

Much had happened in American pharmacy before 1852. Although few trained health care practitioners came with the first settlers to North America, the pioneers came equipped with home medical books and domestic ("kitchen") medicine. As the colonies prospered in the early 1700s, towns grew in size to support businesses such as apothecary shops. In British North America, physicians ran most apothecary shops, combining medical and pharmaceutical practice. The boundaries between medicine and pharmacy were fuzzy at best.

Some eighteenth-century practitioners in the largest cities limited their trade to medicine making and selling. Druggists sold drugs and medicines wholesale to apothecaries, physicians, surgeons, and general store owners. They also dealt in the trade of patent medicines (nostrums), which grew in popularity throughout the 1700s. Almost all the drugs, chemicals, spices, and medicines they sold were imported from England. Few laws applied to pharmacy practice in the Anglo-American colonies and the free market regulated the scene until the 1870s.

The Revolutionary War interrupted trade with England and forced American druggists and apothecaries to obtain their goods through other channels. And while the old trade routes for importation were re-established at war's end, the young United States did have in place a domestic network for the packaging and distribution of drugs and medicines. Most pharmacy, i.e., the compounding of medicines, was still done by physicians in their own

*Gregory J. Higby, PhD, is director, American Institute of the History of Pharmacy.

"doctor's shops" or by their apprentices. The number of non-medical practitioners of pharmacy was small and without a sense of group identity.

Change came to the American pharmaceutical enterprise in the early 1800s. Physicians in larger numbers attended medical schools and gained clinical experience in hospitals and dispensaries rather than with individual preceptors. In these settings, they learned to write out prescriptions for apothecaries to compound and dispense, thereby stimulating the growth of pharmacy. Indicative of this development was the publication of the Massachusetts Pharmacopoeia in 1808 as a state guide to drug standards. It defined the identity of drugs and preparations so that apothecaries could properly fill the prescriptions of physicians. A national convention of physicians authorized the first *Pharmacopoeia of the United States of America* in 1820.

The appearance of these books reflected both the growing amount of prescription writing and the medical profession's increasing reliance on pharmacists. The number of pharmacy practitioners in urban areas reached the critical mass necessary for the establishment of local organizations such as the Philadelphia College of Pharmacy (1821) and the Massachusetts College of Pharmacy (1823). These colleges (the term being used in the sense of associated colleagues) established night schools for the instruction of apprentices and discussion groups on scientific pharmacy. It was an exciting time with alkaloidal chemistry adding new potent drugs to the materia medica. The young American pharmaceutical industry, which arose during the War of 1812 with Great Britain, quickly turned to meet the demands for new products.

Between 1820 and 1860 the boundaries of practice between physicians and pharmacists were drawn. East Coast apothecary shops became more standardized in their appearance and in the stock they carried. Pharmacy followed the trend of specialty retailing and concentrated on drugs, medicines, surgical supplies, artificial teeth and limbs, dyestuffs, essences, and chemicals. Grocers took over the selling of exotic dietary items such as figs, raisins, and citrus fruits. Drugstores in small cities and towns, however, tended to keep in stock more general articles such as glass, paints, varnishes, and oils. Above all, apothecary shops became the main distributors of patent medicines, one of the most profitable lines of merchandise in the history of American business.

Relations between physicians and pharmacists were generally good during the 1830s. Physicians welcomed the early pharmacy colleges and served as faculty in their schools. They supported the independent occupation of pharmacy as a necessary division of labor in a developing society.

The relationship between physicians and pharmacists deteriorated in the 1840s. Feeling more confident of their social standing, apothecaries shifted their efforts from pleasing physicians to attending to the ills of customers. Consequently, American apothecaries took to refilling prescriptions without physician authorization and directly treating customers, a practice called counter-prescribing. In the large cities, doctor's shops were back on the rise after a decline of two decades. Medical schools turned out graduates by the hundreds, most of whom sought their fortunes in urban areas, where they would open shop. Physicians and pharmacists competed directly and sometimes with open hostility.

America had become the dumping ground for the poor quality drugs of

Europe. While it had been common since colonial days for exporters to send shoddy goods overseas, the situation worsened in the 1840s. The drug market within Europe tightened up through regulation. Moreover, the emergence of alkaloidal chemistry made it possible to extract quinine or other alkaloids from medicinal plants and then send the partially (or fully) exhausted bark or root off to America.

The young American Medical Association, working with the local medical and pharmaceutical societies in New York City, helped push through the Drug Importation Act of 1848. The law called for the appointment of special examiners at six major ports of entry—New York, Boston, Philadelphia, Baltimore, Charleston, and New Orleans. Each inspector would check for "quality, purity, and fitness for medical purposes" using the major pharmacopoeias and dispensatories, including the USP, for standards. Although the new law worked well initially, political cronyism soon filled most of the inspector posts with incompetents.

In order to battle this situation, a convention of pharmacists was called together in New York City in 1851. The organizers hoped that a firm set of standards for purity would be approved by the convention for use by the inspectors. The Philadelphia delegation, led by William Procter, Jr., went to New York with an additional agendum in mind—the establishment of a national pharmacy organization. Both were accomplished: the convention came up with a set of standards and called for a national convention to meet in Philadelphia the next year, which resulted in the American Pharmaceutical Association.

When APhA met in 1852, the young organization discussed nine ambitious objectives:

- Create a national association with a constitution and code of ethics;
- Support schools of pharmacy;
- Improve the selection and training of pharmacy apprentices;
- Investigate secret medicines and quackery;
- Urge enactment of laws for the inspection of imported drugs;
- Adopt a National Pharmacopeia as a guide in preparing medicines;
- Curb indiscriminate sale of poisons;
- Separate pharmacy from the practice of medicine;
- Encourage presentation of original papers on pharmacy and science.

All were enormous challenges at a time when there existed no state regulation of pharmacy and just a handful of isolated local pharmaceutical societies and schools. Yet, the APhA met all of these objectives, some after decades of dedicated struggle. The essays in this book celebrate these achievements and point toward the continuing progress of American pharmacy.

Sources

Higby G. Evolution of Pharmacy. In: Gennaro AR, ed. *Remington: The Science and Practice of Pharmacy*, Baltimore: Lippincott Williams & Wilkins; 2000: 11-13.

Higby G. Drug Quality and the Origins of the APhA: The 1851 Convention of Pharmaceutists and Druggists. *J Am Pharm Assoc.* 2002; 42:831-835.

Griffenhagen G, ed. *150 Years of Caring: A Pictorial History of the American Pharmaceutical Association*, Washington, DC: APhA, 2002:6-7.

American Pharmacy's First Great Transformation: Practice, 1852-1902

*by Gregory J. Higby**

LOOKING back from today it is easy to lump together all nineteenth-century pharmacy practice. Perhaps we imagine an 1890s drugstore with mahogany furnishings and shiny soda fountain fixtures. Or we may envision old "doc," the friendly pharmacist, behind the counter ready to dispense remedies for the minor ailments of everyday life. These stereotypes have a great deal of truth behind them, but they tend to hide the enormous changes that enveloped pharmacy practice in the second half of the 1800s. In no other period has pharmacy practice changed so much, including our own. Put simply, a large part of the original raison d'être for the profession in the United States disappeared and the basic role of the pharmacist shifted dramatically.[1]

Although apothecary shops had existed since the founding days of the North American colonies, the classic American drugstore did not appear until the early 1800s. Until then, physicians or their apprentices compounded and dispensed most medications directly to patients.[2] Changes in medical education, the introduction of new drugs, and shifts in the physician-patient relationship during the 1820s and 1830s resulted in the establishment of the drugstore as an American institution.[3] By 1850, a typical American drugstore combined a "front end" composed of a pharmacy work area and general emporium with a miniature factory in the back for making the scores of preparations and ingredients destined to be combined into medicines prescribed by physicians. The proprietor of the shop—the apothecary—supervised a staff of clerks (employed pharmacists) and apprentices who waited on customers and did most of the hard labor of sorting, grinding, sifting, macerating, or filtering the crude drugs that were processed into the products described in the *United States Pharmacopeia*. In this way they learned the science and art

---

*Gregory J. Higby, PhD, is director, American Institute of the History of Pharmacy.

of pharmacy, which they would pass on to their own apprentices. They also learned the ways of the shopkeeper.[4]

When pharmacists gathered in Philadelphia in 1852 to found the American Pharmaceutical Association (APhA), the occupation stood at a crossroads. Its stature, gained through demonstrating the utility of the careful manufacture of drugs and compounding of medications, appeared threatened by a set of problems: Nostrums or quack remedies promising sure cures were being sold everywhere, endangering the public health. The supply of drugs to pharmacies was increasingly adulterated. Poisons were being sold indiscriminately by many persons ignorant of their dangers. No effective laws governed the medical or pharmaceutical professions. And the apprenticeship system for training young apothecaries was starting to break down with the onset of large-scale manufacture of ready-made pharmaceuticals.[5]

At the 1854 APhA meeting William Procter stated, "The larger-number of those who deal in drugs and medicines do so solely to make money; they aim at making the most of the least outlay of capital and trouble. To sell medicines is their vocation."[6] The idea of selling as the center of pharmacy practice outraged Procter. To him and other professionally minded apothecaries, the making of medicines was the heart of pharmacy. Yet, even in 1854, Procter and his allies within the Association battled against the growing tendency of most apothecaries to buy pharmaceutical preparations "ready made" from large manufacturers. Throughout the rest of the century, pharmacy's leaders railed against this shortcut, to no avail.[7]

Soon after the founding of the Association, its members faced an onslaught of professional challenges. Financial crisis at the end of the 1850s slowed commerce and closed the doors of hundreds of drugstores. The Civil War ripped the nation apart and brought most business to a standstill. One beneficiary of the fighting was the young pharmaceutical industry, which burgeoned during the conflict of the 1860s. E. R. Squibb and his competitors scaled up the production of preparations for the war effort and carried these techniques ahead in peacetime. With most basic preparations now available from drug companies, anyone with enough nerve and capital could open up a drugstore. The number of pharmacists grew enormously, and the quality of prescriptions dispensed declined accordingly.[4]

In response to public and professional concern, effective state laws regulating pharmacy were enacted in the 1870s and 1880s. And though the educational infrastructure lagged at first behind the new regulations, the quality of pharmacy practice began to improve. State boards of pharmacy examined prospective pharmacists to ensure minimum competence. An influx of new state-affiliated pharmacy schools in the 1880s and 1890s helped to raise the level of practice significantly.[8]

The passage of laws helped to solidify the professional boundaries between pharmacy and medicine. In the early decades of the nineteenth century, physicians often operated drugstores ("doctor's shops") where they practiced both medicine and pharmacy. At the same time, apothecaries commonly diagnosed and prescribed for customers ("counter-prescribing"). For the leaders of the young APhA, pharmacy's hope as a profession rested on the clear distinction between medical and pharmaceutical practice. The division between the professions during the Civil War helped draw this line. By encouraging this trend, the Association played an important part in pharmacy's progress.[4,5]

New and more effective drugs entered the scene in the late 1800s, including synthetics such as antipyrine, acetanilid, phenacetin, and chloral hydrate. Greater uniformity came to galenical preparations as well, pushed forward by the modernization of the *United States Pharmacopeia*. Large-scale manufacturers took over the making of almost all ingredients by the late 1800s and began moving into the production of end dosage forms as well.[9] The emphasis of pharmacy practice shifted away from manufacturing. Instead, pharmacists stressed their skills as master compounders: Only they could put together the "tailor-made" prescriptions written by physicians to meet the special needs of individual patients. (Typically, these prescriptions called for the combination of one to four active ingredients and a liquid vehicle, which was dispensed in a corked bottle with a label containing the shop's name, the patient's name, and directions for use.)[10]

Unfortunately, Americans continued to turn to secret remedies or cure-alls for their ills. Some physicians had even begun prescribing them for their patients instead of writing out detailed prescriptions. This outraged pharmacists because this practice both encouraged quackery and robbed them of business. To combat this trend, the APhA in 1888 published the first *National Formulary* in the hope that this collection of recipes would encourage the prescribing of medicines that could be easily compounded with standard ingredients from the USP. Although warmly received by physicians and pharmacists alike, the NF could not hold off the trend toward the prescribing of ready-made preparations. It was nearly impossible for the pharmacist on the corner to make up coated pills and complex mixtures with the elegance of the large companies.[11]

Perhaps nothing else influenced everyday pharmacy practice more than the general introduction of mass-produced compressed tablets in the 1890s. By 1902, one young woman in a factory could run a pair of machines punching out one million headache tablets a day. Compounding, the crux of professional practice in the late nineteenth century, started its great decline.

Changes in practice and technology also altered the face of the pharmacy. In 1852, pharmacists put their compounding areas near the front of their shops to benefit from the natural light coming through the windows and to demonstrate their professional abilities. By the 1890s, stores were rearranged, with the prescription table moved to the back of the shop (in place of the laboratory). This opened up the front for high markup goods such as tobacco products and candy. Above all else, the shift of pharmacy practice to the back of the shop gave the soda fountain the front-and-center position. Ironically, it was the pharmacist's expertise that allowed him to make up fresh flavorings and to handle temperamental carbonated water generators. Unfortunately, the public soon came to see pharmacists more as sellers of chocolate sodas than health care professionals.[12]

Conclusion

In 1852 there were no telephones, no typewriters, no automobiles, no laws regulating practice, no state boards of pharmacy, less than a handful of pharmacy schools, and only one (local) pharmacy journal published in North America. By 1902, pharmacies had telephones, typewriters, electric lights, and pharmacists were licensed by state boards and could subscribe to several national journals. Prospective pharmacists had more than 80 pharmacy schools of varying quality from which to choose for their education.

From 1852 to 1902 pharmacists evolved from small manufacturers into compounding experts, and had begun their further transformation into professionalized dispensers. School of pharmacy diplomas and registration certificates gave legitimacy to their professional claims. But as retail practice became more commercialized and less challenging scientifically, many ambitious pharmacists turned to new practice opportunities in hospitals, industry, and academia. The vast majority of pharmacists who remained in retail practice during the next 50 years fought an uphill battle to gain full professional stature while searching for a new role in health care.

This article originally appeared in *Journal of the American Pharmaceutical Association,* (Jan/Feb 2000).

References

1. Higby G. From Compounding to Caring. In: Knowlton CH, Penna RP, eds. *Pharmaceutical Care*, New York: Chapman and Hall; 1995:18-45.
2. Hazen E. *Popular Technology; or Professions and Trades*, New York: Harper and Bros.; 1841.
3. Kilmer FB, Deshler CD. Drug clerks one hundred years ago. *J Am Pharm Assoc.* 1929;18:711-22.
4. Higby G. *In Service to American Pharmacy, the Professional Life of William Procter, Jr.,* Tuscaloosa: University of Alabama Press; 1992.
5. Hoffmann F. A Retrospect of the Development of American Pharmacy and the American Pharmaceutical Association. *Proc Am Pharm Assoc.* 1902;50:100-45.
6. Procter W. An address to the pharmacists of the United States.Proc *Am Pharm Assoc.* 1854; 3:14-22.
7. Remington J. Pharmacy during the last fifty years. *Druggists Circular.* 1907;51:19-25.
8. Higby G. A brief look at American pharmaceutical education before 1900. *Am J Pharm Ed.* 1999; 63S:1-16.
9. Schieffelin WJ. The advances made in pharmaceutical manufactures during the past fifty years. *Proc Am Pharm Assoc.* 1902;50:146-51.
10. Remington J. *Practice of Pharmacy.* Philadelphia: J. B. Lippincott; 1894.
11. Rusby HH. Fifty years of Materia Medica. *Druggists Circular.* 1907;51:29-43.
12. Higby G. Professionalism and the Nineteenth-Century American Pharmacist. *Pharmacy in History.* 1986; 28:115-24.

The American Practice of Pharmacy, 1902-1952

by Glenn Sonnedecker*

B_Y September 8, 1902, more than 500 pharmacists from across the country had arrived at Philadelphia's Hotel Walton for the 50th Annual Meeting of the American Pharmaceutical Association (APhA). Horse-drawn carriages and drays—steering clear of an occasional Stanley Steamer or Oldsmobile—shuttled the conventioneers from the railway station to the celebrative sessions. APhA membership (c. 1,404) had increased to about 3% of the number identified in the latest census as retail "dealers" in "drugs and medicines." Members could take some satisfaction in the professional gains made during the first half-century of their organized effort.[1] But the traditions they prized were being rudely pushed aside by the transforming currents of technologic and economic change.

The Practitioners

For most pharmacists during APhA's second half-century, the drugstore provided full-time employment, but only a part-time practice of pharmacy. Yet the opportunities appealed to American youths who liked the prospect of owning a small-business enterprise combined with the craft and mystique of drug lore. Early in the century the lack of a college requirement also had some appeal to those hard pressed for time or cash. A store-trained apprentice could qualify as a pharmacist by state examination. But a new time and a higher level of practice were on the horizon when, in 1905, New York State began to require graduation from at least a 2-year course in pharmacy. Gradually, one state after another followed suit. By mid-century most newly licensed pharmacists held a 4-year degree, but increasing the practice requirements had been a stepwise, erratic process among the states. Partial 1947

*Glenn Sonnedecker, PhD, is professor-emeritus, School of Pharmacy, University of Wisconsin-Madison, and director-emeritus, American Institute of the History of Pharmacy. Illustrations were reproduced with the kind permission of the F. B. Power Pharmaceutical Library, University of Wisconsin-Madison, and the American Institute of the History of Pharmacy (Drug Topics Collection).

data, for example, suggest the following alloca-
tion among 20 practitioners: 5 nongraduates; 6
two-year graduates; 3 three-year graduates; and
6 four-year graduates.[2]

An uncontrolled growth in personnel, and
in the Anglo-American spirit of free enterprise
spawned intense competition (especially in urban areas) as well as opportunity. Between 1900
and 1948 the number of active pharmacists grew
from an estimated 57,000 to about 90,000, although the effect was blunted by a doubling of
the U.S. population. The number of women
pharmacists also increased, from about 2% of
American pharmacists to nearly 5%.[3]

At least half of all pharmacists were owners or managers of the establishment in which
they worked, in a triple role as proprietor, professional pharmacist, and general salesperson.
At mid-century, 52% of the drugstores were still
serviced by a single pharmacist with the long
hours that implied.[4] An unsatisfactory response
to the need for assistance was the authorization
of "assistant pharmacists" in about nine-tenths
of the states. These second-class practitioners—
whose only licensure qualification was, variably,
1 to 4 years of drugstore experience—could ful-
fill (under supervision) the duties of a registered
pharmacist, even in the "temporary absence" of
the latter. By 1926 about 20,000 assistant pharmacists were behind drugstore counters.

So many questions of usurped responsibilities and substandard services emerged from
this arrangement that by the 1930s state legislatures began to revoke authorization for the licensing of more assistant pharmacists. By mid-century only
1,336 remained in practice, and this divisive personnel issue gradually drew
to a close.[5]

*Facade of a small-town
drugstore in Wisconsin,
early 20th century. Typi-
cal display windows fea-
ture colorful showglobes
and product promotions.
Townsfolk far down Main
Street were reminded of
the pharmacy by the giant
wooden mortar projecting
over the sidewalk.*

The Drugstore

Although the size and character of drugstores varied greatly, most
pharmacists could expect commercial and professional duties to compete
for their time. Pressure from competition and from higher state standards
gradually reduced the number of shops in relation to the population during
the first half of the 20th century, moving from about 2,030 citizens per drugstore in 1903 to 3,140 in 1948.

An unexpected challenge to independent pharmacies arose from a general trend toward combining retail enterprises into chains. Around the turn
of the century—perhaps influenced by earlier British combinations—an occasional pharmacist-entrepreneur was linking several drugstores together
under a single ownership. The implications of absentee ownership for the

traditional "corner druggist" became clearer when Charles R. Walgreen acquired 116 drugstores between 1901 and 1927 and Louis K. Liggett acquired 672 drugstores between 1907 and 1930. The chain store's expanded sidelines, innovative self-service, and aggressive mass-merchandising strategy took the commercialization of retail pharmacy to a new level. Traditions of the American drugstore rendered it vulnerable to the business efficiencies and practices of chain operation, and independent owners were apprehensive at mid-century that this urban phenomenon could affect pharmacy even further.[6] Independent pharmacists also felt beleaguered by competition from new departments in supermarkets and department stores.

The Medications Dispensed

The long-range trend of the period was toward expanded prescription practice, a near disappearance of the compounding function, and a revolution in drug therapy. The amount of compounding had continued to drop. A 1920 survey suggested that almost 80% of prescription orders still required "some" compounding; by the late 1940s, however, it was about 26%, and by 1951 it was down to about 10%.[7]

More encouraging was an upward trend in the number of prescriptions dispensed, although many physicians in rural areas still dispensed ready-made drugs from their offices. A 1930s study indicated that an average drugstore received only eight prescriptions per day. In reality there was a wide variation. For example, probably at least one pharmacy in 100 received a majority of its income from prescriptions, whereas village pharmacies sometimes received only 5 to 10 prescription orders per week. About one-third of these prescriptions specified trade-named or patented products (in the early

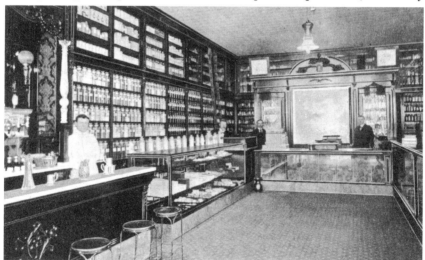

An urban drugstore of 1902 with typical features but superior elegance: prescription department in the rear; shelves laden with matched sets of stock bottles for botanical powders, tinctures, fluid extracts; over-the-counter medications, sickroom supplies, and sundries behind a counter or under glass; and an ornate soda fountain.

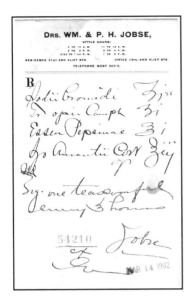

Characteristics of this 1902 pre-scription order were disappearing from practice by 1952: the Latin nomenclature, the apothecaries' system of metrology, the domi-nance of natural products, and polypharmacal prescribing.

1930s).[8] An upsurge in prescription practice (orders tripled for example between 1940 and 1955) was spurred by strikingly more effective therapeutic agents coupled with regulatory changes. Transforming innovations during the half-century included immunologic agents, parenteral medications, the first chemotherapy (arsphenamine and the sulfonamides), antibiotics (penicillin and streptomycin), pure vitamins and hormones, and a breakthrough in psychoactives (chlorpromazine).

Of the estimated total expenditure for medications in drugstores during 1929, prescriptions accounted for about 22%. An additional 24% was spent on generic home remedies of known formula, mostly the so-called "druggists' preparations" that bore a pharmacy's own label. Approximately 54% of medication expenditures in drugstores went for secret-formula nostrums—mass produced and mass promoted to the public—exploiting claims that were often misleading or fraudulent.[9] APhA long opposed such exploitation, but a majority of pharmacists supplied "patent medicines" (rarely actually patented) on grounds of public demand and legality. The worst excesses gradually came under control through laws and regulations enacted between 1906 and 1938 (to be discussed later in this series).

A more benign commercialization of the workplace lay in the ever-changing array of sidelines unrelated to pharmacy, most notably the "soda fountain." Especially after federal enactment of Prohibition (1919), the drugstore fountain became a social center affectionately regarded by youths and adults alike. Within a decade about 60% of American drugstores were operating fountains, and the number grew. More stools were added; tables began to preempt floor space; food service became increasingly important at the cash register. Then, during World War II, fountains began to disappear from drugstores, largely because of a shortage in personnel and a decrease in profit.[6] By the 1950s it appeared that the time when the citizenry no longer identified soda fountain delights with pharmacy seemed imminent.

The Hospital Pharmacy

The different work setting of hospital pharmacists fostered a striking difference in professional development. By the 1920s the national network of hospitals was being upgraded and expanded, influenced in part by the American Hospital Association (founded in 1899) and by a new cadre of professional hospital administrators. Hospital pharmacists had been largely unappreciated and undercompensated, and before the 1930s perhaps three-fourths of the small hospitals (i.e., fewer than 150 beds) employed no pharmacist full-time. Some practitioners began to agitate for a higher level of practice and for institutional recognition of professional standing.

These professional ambitions were harnessed at first through APhA, then through the American Society of Hospital Pharmacists (founded in 1942). Progress was impressive: Practitioners organized local groups; standards for internships in hospital practice were implemented, and graduate instruction fostered; hospital formularies appeared, coupled with a role for the pharmacist as drug therapy consultant to the medical and nursing staffs. More of the ill-equipped pharmacies were upgraded after Congress, in 1947, began to implement the Hospital Survey and Construction Act. Additional stimulus came from the U.S. Public Health Service through its influential "Suggested Plans for Hospital Pharmacies for 50, 100, and 200 Bed General Hospitals" (1950).[10] All this permitted hospital pharmacists to use their professional knowledge to an extent not feasible for the average community pharmacist.

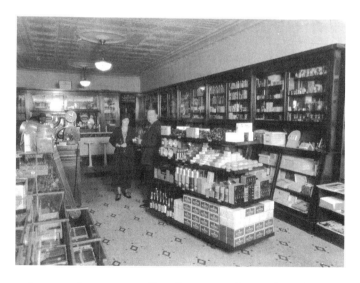

In the early 1930s drugstores ordinarily were no larger than this one in Ohio. Handsome wall cabinets of dark wood were still popular, but the shelving now held trade-named, factory-packaged products—no longer the A-to-Z rows of stock bottles for bulk supplies of medicaments. An island display of sundries now began to encourage self-service.

Harbingers of Change

As APhA approached its Centennial Meeting in 1952, community pharmacists also seemed poised for reform efforts. These focused on implementing the recommendations from a "Pharmaceutical Survey" (1946-1949) that was the most broad-ranging evaluation of American pharmacy up to that time. Meanwhile, APhA was promoting experimental programs during the 1940s in which pharmacists disseminated public health information, pilot projects with themes of venereal disease prevention and warning signs of cancer. To replace the vanishing medicine-making role, some advocated that practitioners reach out as drug therapy consultants to the other health professions. But an occasional call for greater "patient orientation" drew limited response in accord with pharmacy's long-standing ethical requirement that a pharmacist "never discuss the therapeutic effect of a physician's prescription with a patron nor disclose details of composition." Still, some wondered whether a counseling function to help assure the safe and effective use of medications might be a valid social role for future pharmacists.

This article originally appeared in *Journal of the American Pharmaceutical Association,* (Jan/Feb 2001).

References

1. Higby G. American pharmacy's first great transformation: practice, 1852-1902. *J Am Pharm Assoc.* 2000;40:9-10.
2. Elliott EC, ed. *The General Report of the Pharmaceutical Survey 1946-49.* Washington, DC: American Council on Education. 1950:31 (14 to 19 states reported data to NABP). *Proc. Natl. Assoc. Bds. of Pharm.* 1951:47.
3. Census 1900 through *Druggists Circ.*1907; 51(Jan.):151. *Proc. Natl. Assoc. Bds. Pharm.* 1951; 47th Meeting:48. Rorem CR, Fischelis RP. *The Costs of Medicines and the Services of Pharmacists in Medical Care.* Chicago: University of Chicago; c. 1932:33 & 183.
4. *Proc Natl Assoc Bds Pharm* 1951: 57.
5. Ibid.:58 & 75. Beard JG. The assistant pharmacist: a dangerous anomaly. *J Am Pharm Assoc.* 1926; 15:1119-26.
6. Sonnedecker G (revisor). *Kremers and Urdang's History of Pharmacy.* Philadelphia: Lippincott; 1976:297-299. Rorem and Fischelis, n. 3:75 f.
7. Rivera-Gonzalez R. "Prescription Compounding; A Socio-Professional Characterization." MSc thesis, Madison: University of Wisconsin; 1966:24 (citing WW Charters, 1927; JS Mordell, 1949; Abbott Laboratories . . . Survey, 1952).
8. Rorem and Fischelis. n. 3:59 & 69 (fn 9). Gathercoal EN. *The Prescription Ingredient Survey.* . . . n.p.: APhA; 1933:10 & 15.
9. Rorem and Fischelis. n. 3:18, 57, cf. 218. About 7% of the total spent for nostrums in the USA went to non-pharmacy distributors of packaged medicines, thus not included in the drugstore figures mentioned.
10. Niemeyer G, Berman A, Francke DE. *Ten Years of the American Society of Hospital Pharmacists 1942-1952,* republished from the ASHP's Bulletin. 1952; 9: 281-421. See also, Berman A. Historical Currents in American Hospital Pharmacy. *Drug Intelligence & Clin Pharm.* 1972;6: 441-7.

The Continuing Evolution of American Pharmacy Practice, 1952-2002

by Gregory J. Higby*

In 1952 customers left American drugstores with prescription vials absent the name of the drug inside; today, patients leave American pharmacies with fully labeled vials plus pages of medication information. The basic function of pharmacy practice—accurately dispensing prescription orders—remains. Fifty years of professional debate, governmental regulation, and expansion of the role third party payers play, though, have significantly altered the secondary aspects of practice.

Following World War II, American pharmaceutical firms applied cutting-edge technology to the production of medications and rapidly became one of the most advanced industries in the world. New drugs, new dosage forms, and new marketing methods reinforced a trend evident from the early 1900s of physicians shifting away from prescribing complex mixtures of ingredients toward prescribing brand-name ready-made, single-entity medications mass-manufactured by large companies.[1] In the 1930s about 75% of prescriptions required some compounding; by 1950 that figure had dropped below 25%. During the 1950s this decline accelerated until only about 1 in 25 prescriptions required any compounding, bottoming out in 1970 at about 1 in 100.[2]

During the late 1940s, both governmental agencies and pharmacy groups struggled with ways to regulate the use of dangerous and addictive medications. In 1951 Congressman Carl Durham (D-NC) and Senator Hubert Humphrey (D-MN) put forward an amendment to the 1938 Food, Drug and Cosmetic Act that more clearly defined a prescription drug. Although organized pharmacy argued for a third class of medications to be available through pharmacies only, the amendment defined just two—what became

---

*Gregory J. Higby, PhD, is director, American Institute of the History of Pharmacy, School of Pharmacy, University of Wisconsin-Madison.

known as prescription "legend" drugs and over-the-counter (OTC) medications. The new amendment effectively removed the discretionary power that pharmacists had over the sale of drugs.

The Era of Count and Pour

The restricted nature of postwar practice is reflected in the APhA Code of Ethics of 1952: "The pharmacist does not discuss the therapeutic effects or composition of a prescription with a patient. When such questions are asked he suggests that the qualified practitioner [i.e., physician or dentist] is the proper person with whom such matters should be discussed."[3] The era of "count and pour" pharmacy had begun in community practice. (Hospital pharmacy practice also concentrated on the product but was more varied, as

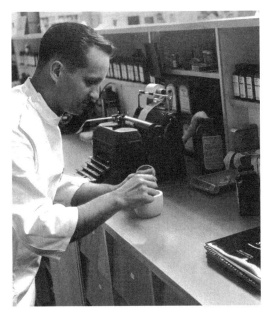

In the 1930s, 75% of prescriptions were compounded. This number dropped below 25% in the 1950s. By the 1970s pharmacists compounded only 1 in every 100 prescriptions. This photograph shows a pharmacist at work in Roseville Drive-In Drug Co., Roseville, Michigan, in 1956.

hospital pharmacists dealt with issues of large-scale compounding, distribution within institutions, and pharmacy and therapeutics [P&T] committees.[4])

The 1950s were marked by unprecedented growth in the number of new drug products. Of the thousands of medications introduced, many were duplicates. In 1952, 45 oral penicillin preparations were being produced by 17 companies. For efficiency and standardization of care, hospitals developed formulary systems that allowed pharmacists to dispense generic equivalents in place of brand-name products. Pharmaceutical manufacturers fought hard to prevent substitution in both community and institutional settings. A manufacturers' trade group, the National Pharmaceutical Council, succeeded in getting states to pass laws forbidding the replacement of a prescribed brand-name product with a generic product. Community pharmacists protested but followed the new laws. Prescription volume was rising rapidly and becoming the financial engine of most American drugstores. On the hospital front, however, pharmacists resisted, and they worked throughout the 1950s to devise systems that allowed for generic product selection. By the 1960s blanket prior-consent procedures allowed hospitals to operate formularies more efficiently.[5, 6]

Clinical Pharmacy Emerges

Looking back, the 1960s seem to have been years of revolution. No revolt occurred in pharmacy, but the forces of reform did bring changes. And, as with other grassroots movements, the push to change clinical pharmacy came from everyday people—pharmacy practitioners. In 1960 a pharmacist named Eugene V. White remodeled his Berryville, VA, drugstore into an office-style practice and started using patient profile cards. In 1965 APhA promoted a Pharmaceutical Center based on White's ideas. Although the center never displaced the traditional American drugstore, its design influenced consultation areas throughout U.S. pharmacies.[7]

The major impetus for clinical pharmacy came from the institutional sector of practice. For most of American history, hospital pharmacy was seen as a secondary part of the profession, as being beneath the pinnacle of store ownership and retail practice. Beginning in the 1920s, however, a new camaraderie arose among hospital practitioners. As manufacturing, and then compounding, disappeared from community pharmacy, hospital pharmacists continued to use their expertise. During the 1940s and 1950s, as new, potent drug products appeared on the market, hospital pharmacists gained

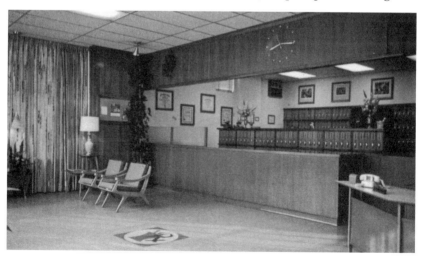

APhA unveiled the "Pharmaceutical Center" at its 1965 Annual Meeting based on a concept developed by Eugene V. White of Berryville, VA (shown above). U.S. Vice President Hubert H. Humphrey and McKesson & Robbins Chairman of the Board Herman Nolan cut the ribbon to open the center, which was named after APhA's first president, Daniel B. Smith.

more control over these products. P&T committees and hospital formularies granted pharmacy a voice in therapeutic decisions. A team of hospital pharmacists led by Don Francke surveyed the status of institutional practice and published their results in the landmark 1964 work *Mirror to Hospital Pharmacy*.[8] The scene was set for pharmacists to become therapeutic advisors.

By the mid-1960s, Donald Brodie was arguing that "the ultimate goal of the services of pharmacy must be the safe use of drugs by the public. In this context, the mainstream function of pharmacy is clinical in nature, one that may be identified accurately as drug-use control . . . i.e., the sum total of knowledge, understanding, judgments, procedures, skills, controls, and ethics that assures optimal safety in the distribution and use of medication."[9] This more aggressive approach to practice was adopted by others, such as the famous ninth-floor project at the University of California-San Francisco. Initiated in 1966, this project pioneered uses of several components essential to modern hospital pharmacy practice, such as technicians, unit dose, patient drug profiles, and a drug information center.[10] As the utility of clinical pharmacy was demonstrated, institutions across the nation expanded their pharmacy departments. During the 1970s and 1980s, hospital staff pharmacists more than doubled to nearly one fourth of all practitioners.[11]

Pharmacy's general adoption of the ideals of clinical pharmacy is evident in the 1969 Code of Ethics of APhA. Rather than being advised to hide behind the authority of physicians, practitioners of pharmacy were told boldly, "A pharmacist should . . . render to each patient the full measure of his ability as an essential health practitioner."[12] Writing in 1970, Melvin R. Gibson put forward the profession's new confidence: "The pharmacist is the only expert on drugs. . . . No educational program other than that in pharmacy provides the background to completely understand all there is to understand about drugs. The pharmacist, and the pharmacist alone, is in that unique position of embracing complete drug expertise."[13]

Rank-and-file pharmacists gradually adopted the role of drug advisor. Customers had traditionally relied on the advice of pharmacists concerning minor ailments and came to ask more and more about their prescriptions. Released from previous restrictions, pharmacists came to view the people across the counter as patients rather than customers. Rudimentary profile systems gave pharmacists a tool for checking compliance and preventing interactions. The evolution of practice had begun.

The establishment of Medicare and Medicaid in 1965 changed the pharmaceutical landscape significantly. Medicare stimulated the growth of hospital practice by requiring pharmacist directors for reimbursement.[6] Medicaid brought millions of new prescriptions into community pharmacies—along with the resulting headaches of paperwork, reimbursement hassles, and regulation.[14]

The burgeoning of third party programs, both through private insurance and government support, created an exploding demand for pharmaceutical services. The high cost of prescription drugs stimulated government agencies to study cost-cutting approaches, including generic substitution. In 1970 the APhA House of Delegates advocated the repeal of antisubstitution laws, and a year later APhA published a white paper titled the "Pharmacist's Role in Product Selection," which argued the case.[15] The consumer movement of the 1970s helped secure the repeal of these laws, which started with Michigan in 1974. Cost savings came slowly, however, as pharmacists were initially reluctant to substitute.[16] Another cost-containment measure instituted was the Health Maintenance Organization Act of 1973, which opened the era of managed care.

Computerization

In the late 1970s keyboards and monitors entered prescription departments across the United States. The early computer systems were expensive and low on power, but they offered pharmacists a solution for dealing with the mountains of paperwork piling up in pharmacy back rooms. Problems with Medicaid were notorious, and, although the first computers were far from flawless, they brought a higher degree of accuracy to the payment system. As prices dropped on hardware and as software became more sophisticated in the 1980s, pharmacists adopted computers as quickly as members of any profession. They soon learned how to check for drug interactions and track profiles to improve patient care.[17]

The decade of the 1980s was dominated by the presidency of economic conservative Ronald Reagan. In the climate of wide-open capitalism, mass marketers such as Wal-Mart built superstores in small towns across America, forcing out many independent pharmacies. And mail service pharmacy, which had been a tiny part of the industry for decades, grew into a force.[5] During the 1980s both private companies and governmental agencies adopted the practices of managed care. By the middle of the 1990s, two-thirds of Americans got their health care through a plan connected with managed care.[18] The eventual impact on pharmacy practice was enormous; pharmacists were often caught between patients and managed care organizations (MCOs). An entire new industry, pharmacy benefits management (PBM) firms, arose to

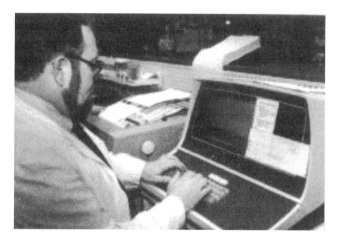

In 1980 fewer than 3,000 community pharmacies were using computer automation to assist in the dispensing function. By 1985 computers were well on their way to becoming an essential tool for a broad range of pharmacy functions.

meet the needs of MCOs struggling to deal with the complex nature of pharmacy services.[18]

During the 1980s, in the midst of economic and scientific change, the leaders of the profession gathered in a series of conferences dedicated to charting a future course for pharmacy. At the second Pharmacy in the 21st Century Conference in 1989, C. Douglas Hepler and Linda Strand proposed a new practice paradigm they labeled "pharmaceutical care."[5] Pharmaceutical care called for pharmacists to take responsibility for drug use control "leading to specific therapeutic outcomes."[19] Even in the midst of the managed care crunch, with economic issues confronting all segments of pharmacy, the leaders of the pharmacy profession enthusiastically adopted the establishment of pharmaceutical care as the profession's primary goal in the decade ahead.[20]

Aspects of pharmaceutical care were included in the Omnibus Budget Reconciliation Act of 1990 (OBRA '90), which "recognized pharmacists as professionals whose expertise can be effectively utilized to . . . promote rational outcomes from drug therapy."[21] The regulations of OBRA '90 called for mandatory drug utilization review for Medicaid recipients and for pharmacists to offer counseling to these patients.[22]

The 1990s were envisioned by many as the dawning of the Pharmaceutical Care Era. Instead, the decade witnessed the consolidation of the pharmaceutical enterprise, with widespread closure of independent pharmacies and mergers galore in the manufacturing and chain sectors. In the face of the Clinton administration's efforts to reform health care, the industry had retrenched. In reaction to burgeoning costs, third party payers (government agencies, insurers, and PBMs) clamped down, using restrictive formularies, generic incentives, and other techniques. With new, effective drugs on the market to treat the problems of a graying population, prescription volume skyrocketed. The end result was that pharmacists were generally too busy dispensing and meeting the cost-controlling measures of MCOs to devote much time to providing pharmaceutical care. Although studies had shown it to be cost-effective practice, only a few programs were initiated for the reimbursement of pharmaceutical care services.[23]

At the beginning of the 21st century, American pharmacists are uncertain about the nature of their future practice. Innovations introduced in recent years, including specialization, automation, certified technicians, and cybertechnology, should facilitate an expansion of pharmacists' professional roles. Yet, the explosive growth in the demand for core pharmacy functions— accurate dispensing and provision of drug information—plus the concomitant administrative workload imposed by managed care has overwhelmed the current workforce.[24] Despite greater opportunities for some practitioners to provide pharmaceutical care in certain settings, most pharmacists are still limited primarily to performing distributive tasks. Their practice is an amalgam of aspects of count and pour pharmacy, drug information (clinical pharmacy), a tincture of pharmaceutical care, and a large amount of managed care wrangling. It may be that a new mixture of pharmacy services will arise from today's models and eventually supersede pharmaceutical care.[4, 25]

The evolution of American pharmacy practice continues.

This article originally appeared in *Journal of the American Pharmaceutical Association* (Jan/Feb 2002).

References

1. Sonnedecker G. The American practice of pharmacy, 1902-1952. *J Am Pharm Assoc.* 2001;41:21-3.
2. Higby GJ. Evolution of pharmacy. In: *Gennaro AR, ed. Remington: The Science and Practice of Pharmacy.* Baltimore, Md: Lippincott; 2000: 7-18.
3. Buerki RA, Vottero LV. *Ethical Responsibility in Pharmacy Practice.* Madison, WI: American Institute of the History of Pharmacy; 1994:155.
4. Holland RW, Nimmo CM. Transitions, part 1: beyond pharmaceutical care. *Am J Health Syst Pharm.* 1999;56:1758 64.
5. Higby GJ. American pharmacy in the twentieth century. *Am J Health Syst Pharm.* 1997;54:1805 15.
6. Harris RR, McConnell WE. The American Society of Hospital Pharmacists: a history. *Am J Hosp Pharm.* 1993; 50(suppl 2):S1-3.
7. Gibson MR. Pharmacists in practice. In: *Remington's Pharmaceutical Sciences.* 14th ed. Easton, Pa: Mack 1970:29.
8. Francke DE. *Mirror to Hospital Pharmacy.* Washington, DC: American Society of Hospital Pharmacists; 1964.
9. Brodie DC, Benson RA. The evolution of the clinical pharmacy concept. *Drug Intell Clin Pharm.* 1976;10:507.
10. Smith WE. The future role of the hospital pharmacist in the patient care area. *Am J Hosp Pharm.* 1967;24:22-31.
11. *Pharmacy Manpower Project State and National Survey Reports.* Ann Arbor, Mich: Vector Research; 1993.
12. Buerki RA, Vottero LV. *Ethical Responsibility in Pharmacy Practice.* Madison, Wis: American Institute of the History of Pharmacy; 1994 158.
13. Gibson MR. Scope of pharmacy. In: *Remington's Pharmaceutical Sciences.* 14th ed. Easton, Pa: Mack; 1970.3.
14. McCarthy RL. Schafermeyer KW. *Introduction to Health Care Delivery: A Primer for Pharmacists.* Gaithersburg, Md: Aspen Publishers; 2001: 67.
15. The pharmacist's role in product selection. *J Am Pharm Assoc.* 1971;NS11:181-99.
16. Ascione FJ, Kirking DM, Gaither CA, Welage LS. Historical overview of generic medication policy. *J Am Pharm Assoc.* 2001;41:567-77.
17. 20 years of pharmacy automation: then and now. *ComputerTalk.* 1997,17(5): 20-9.
18. *The Changing Health Care System: Fostering Relationships Between Managed Care and Pharmacy.* Washington, DC: American Pharmaceutical Association; 1996:4.
19. Hepler CD, Strand LM. Opportunities and responsibilities in pharmaceutical care. *Am J Hosp Pharm.* 1990;47:533-43.
20. Maine LL, Penna RP. Pharmaceutical care—an overview. In: Knowlton CH, Penna RP, eds. *Pharmaceutical Care.* New York NY: Chapman & Hall; 1995:133-54.
21. Brushwood DB, Catizone CA, Coster JM. OBRA '90: what it means to your practice. *US. Pharmacist.* October 1992: 64-72.
22. Gebhart F. Is OBRA '90 working? *Drug Topics.* January 1998:5-60, 63, 65.
23. West DS, Herbert DA, Knowlton CH. The practice of community pharmacy. In: Gennaro AR, ed. *Remington: The Science and Practice of Pharmacy.* Baltimore, Md: Lippincott; 2000: 28-32.
24. Mott DA, Sorofman BA, Kreling DH, et al. A four-state summary of the pharmacy workforce. *J Am Pharm Assoc.* 2001;41:693-702.
25. Hepler CD. Philosophical issues raised by pharmaceutical care. *J Pharm Teaching.* 1996;5(1-2):44.

The Pharmaceutical Sciences in America, 1852-1902

*by John Parascandola**

T HE second half of the 19th century was a period of revolutionary change in the biomedical sciences. The development of the germ theory of disease and the establishment of fields such as bacteriology, pharmacology, and physiological chemistry laid the groundwork for significant advances in medicine and pharmacy. The extraordinary growth of the biomedical sciences also made its impact felt on medical and pharmaceutical education.[1]

Science in Pharmacy Education

The amount and level of science in the pharmaceutical curriculum in the United States before the Civil War was not very high. Glenn Sonnedecker has concluded, for example, that the materia medica and pharmacy lectures in this period often had "little scientific content, in the sense of the theoretic and systematic study of natural phenomena relating to the various phases of pharmacy."[2] In Sonnedecker's view, chemistry formed the scientific core of early American pharmaceutical education. In fact, he went so far as to say that, "for a long time chemistry was the only subject taught in American pharmacy schools that can even be called scientific." Nevertheless, even chemistry was taught only through lectures. There was no laboratory instruction in any of the subjects taught in American pharmacy schools before the Civil War.[3]

It was not until pharmacy schools began to become affiliated with state universities, beginning in the 1860s, that science came to play a much more important role in pharmaceutical education. The pharmacy program established at the University of Michigan in 1868, under the leadership of physician-chemist Albert Prescott, made the study of pharmacy essentially a full-time occupation for the 2 years of the curriculum. It also introduced extensive laboratory training in the basic sciences. Other schools of pharmacy eventually adopted this model, beginning with the University of Wisconsin,

*John Parascandola, PhD, is the former Public Health Service Historian, Department of Health and Human Services.

which established its pharmacy program in 1883.

Wisconsin lured a first-rate pharmaceutical scientist to head its program. Frederick B. Power graduated from the Philadelphia College of Pharmacy in 1874 and earned a PhD in 1880 from the University of Strassburg in Germany. Power remained at Wisconsin for 10 years, establishing the pharmacy curriculum on a firm scientific footing and beginning a tradition of scientific research in the pharmacy program through his own investigations in phytochemistry. His successor, Edward Kremers, continued and even expanded upon the scientific direction that Power had given the program.[4]

Glenn Sonnedecker has examined the experimental work associated with American schools of pharmacy in the 19th century. In the period before 1870, the vast majority of experimental work of any significance occurred at the Philadelphia College of Pharmacy, with the emphasis being on plant chemistry. With the introduction of pharmacy curricula based more on laboratory science in the last few decades of the century, there was a substantial increase in research activity, especially at the schools associated with state universities. Sonnedecker has concluded, however, that many of the papers resulting from research at the state universities in this period were not obviously related to pharmacy and were not published in pharmaceutical journals. A substantial number of these papers were written by chemists and botanists on the pharmacy faculty, or even by individuals affiliated with the pharmacy school who actually held university chairs in fields such as geology or mineralogy.[5]

A crucial factor in the advance of scientific research in pharmacy schools was the introduction of graduate programs, which did not occur until the 20th century. The first doctoral degree for work in a pharmacy school was

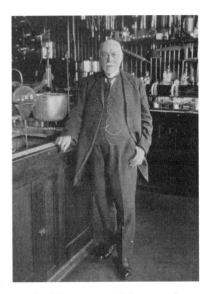

Frederick B. Power (1853-1927), the first director of the University of Wisconsin School of Pharmacy, put scientific research on a firm footing. Power later served as director of the Wellcome Chemical Research Laboratory.

awarded in 1902—at the very end of the period under consideration in this article—at the University of Wisconsin. Even then, however, the degree had to be awarded through the Department of Chemistry, because the Department of Pharmacy did not acquire the administrative authority to grant a PhD degree until 1917.[4]

Chemistry and pharmacognosy dominated the pharmaceutical sciences in colleges of pharmacy at first. Pharmacology was slower to gain a foothold in pharmaceutical education. Courses in pharmacology did not replace materia medica courses until well into the 20th century at most American schools of pharmacy. Although research was carried out on pharmaceutical subjects that we would now consider to be a part of pharmaceutics (such as problems

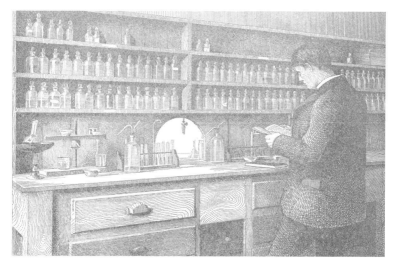

By the 1880s, most U.S. schools of pharmacy had established laboratory experience leading to research activity. This 1889 "chemical laboratory" at the Chicago College of Pharmacy (which subsequently affiliated with the University of Illinois) included 14 sessions of 2 hours each in qualitative chemical analysis.

related to drug delivery), pharmaceutics did not actually become established as a science in this country until about the middle of the 20th century.

Science in the Pharmaceutical Industry

Science also began to enter the American pharmaceutical industry in the second half of the 20th century. With few exceptions, original research remained unorganized and rare in American pharmaceutical companies before the 20th century, as contrasted with the situation in Germany, where research laboratories became common in the major drug firms in the late 19th century. It is true that many of the American companies did establish laboratories in the second half of the 19th century. The goal of these facilities, however, was not research aimed at the development of new drug entities or innovation in general, but rather the standardization of the quantity and quality of ingredients and the potency of existing products. They were largely concerned, in other words, with quality control. Nevertheless, for the first time these firms began to hire chemists, pharmacists, and physicians for analytical work. These analytical laboratories also sometimes became involved in aspects of the control of manufacturing processes.[6]

As Jonathan Liebenau has noted, science was at first more superficial than a driving force in the American pharmaceutical industry. Companies that could promise to deliver standardized preparations had an edge in winning the confidence of the public and the health professions. Thus, in 1861, Parke, Davis and Company hired physician Albert B. Lyons to establish a systematic program of assaying alkaloidal drugs and fluid extracts. In the mid-1880s, Eli Lilly and Company established a Scientific Department, largely an analytical laboratory at first, with pharmacy graduates Josiah K. Lilly and Ernest G. Eberhardt as chemists.[7]

The earliest organized research programs in the American pharmaceutical industry were established in the 1890s by Parke Davis in Detroit and H. K. Mulford Company in Philadelphia in connection with their production of diphtheria antitoxin. Here again, concerns over standardization, in this case biological rather than chemical, were instrumental in persuading the companies to hire staff with expertise in areas such as bacteriology and pharmacology and to establish special laboratories. The scientists who were involved with the production and biological standardization of the antitoxin, however, were soon devoting time to research in new procedures and products. In 1902, once again at the end of the period under consideration in this article, Parke Davis opened what is widely believed to be the first separate building erected by an American drug firm for research.[8]

Science and the American Pharmaceutical Association

The American Pharmaceutical Association (APhA), founded in 1852, also played a role in the development of the pharmaceutical sciences in the United States. One of the original objectives of the Association, as stated in its constitution, was to improve both the art and science of pharmacy by diffusing scientific knowledge, fostering pharmaceutical literature, and encouraging discovery and invention. By the second annual meeting of the organization, scientific papers became an established part of the program and prizes were soon thereafter being offered for the best papers to encourage members to undertake scientific investigations. In 1874 APhA began awarding the Ebert Prize for scientific research, which continues today to be a badge of recognition for significant research contributions to pharmaceutical science.

In 1887 four sections were established within APhA, one of which was the Section on Scientific Papers (renamed the Scientific Section in 1913). In addition to providing a forum for scientific papers at the annual meeting, the Section encouraged research through the awarding of prizes (beginning in 1892, for example, it assumed responsibility for the Ebert Prize).

In George Griffenhagen's analysis of the papers given before the Section on Scientific Papers, he noted that in the years before the Section on Practical Pharmacy was created in 1900, a great many of the papers were concerned with matters of compounding, incompatibilities, drug standards, and the like. In the first 5 years of the Section, about 40% of the papers were devoted to these types of topics. About 30% of the papers in this period could be classified as pharmacognosy, and another 25% as pharmaceutical chemistry.[9]

Griffenhagen's analysis also showed that in the initial 5-year period about half of the papers were contributed by practicing pharmacists who had no association with either industry or a school of pharmacy. It seems fair to assume that most of the papers identified by Griffenhagen as dealing with the more pragmatic topics, such as compounding and incompatibilities, were delivered by practicing pharmacists, who had no venue at the annual meeting to report on their work before the creation of the Section on Practical Pharmacy. Although many practicing pharmacists were carrying out at least rudimentary scientific investigations in the late 19th century, the pharmacy shop did not become a major center for highly significant scientific research. Even in the case of the "Father of American Pharmacy," William Procter, Jr.,

Gregory Higby has concluded that "the quality of Procter's scientific work does not appear exceptional."[10] Unlike Europe, the United States has never produced practicing pharmacist-scientists of the caliber of Carl Scheele or Joseph Pierre Pelletier, who made important discoveries in the laboratories associated with their pharmacies. It should be noted, however, that the sciences were becoming increasingly specialized by the second half of the 19th century, and the tradition of the apothecary-scientist was on the wane even in Europe by this time.

This article originally appeared in *Journal of the American Pharmaceutical Association* 40, no. 6 (Nov/Dec 2000): 733-35.

References

1. Parascandola J. The emergence of pharmaceutical science. *Pharmacy in History.* 1995;37:68-75.
2. Sonnedecker G. Science in American pharmaceutical education of the 19th century. *Am J Pharm Ed.* 1951;15:185-217.
3. Sonnedecker G. The scientific background of chemistry teachers in representative pharmacy schools of the 19th century. *Chymia.* 1953;4:171-200.
4. Sonnedecker G. *Kremers and Urdang's History of Pharmacy.* 4th ed. Philadelphia: J.B. Lippincott; 1976:226-54.
5. Sonnedecker G. Experimental work associated with American pharmaceutical education of the 19th century. In: *Medizingeschichte in unserer Zeit.* Eulner H, Mann G, Preiser G, et al., eds. Stuttgart, Germany: Ferdinand Enke Verlag; 1971:384-92.
6. Weikel M, Sonnedecker G. Emergence of research as a function of the American pharmaceutical industry. Unpublished manuscript (1963). Copy at American Institute of the History of Pharmacy, Madison, Wisc.
7. Liebenau, J. *Medical Science and Medical Technology: The Formation of the American Pharmaceutical Industry.* Baltimore, Md: Johns Hopkins University Press; 1987.
8. Swann J. *Academic Scientists and the Pharmaceutical Industry: Cooperative Research in Twentieth-Century America.* Baltimore, Md: Johns Hopkins University Press; 1988.
9. Griffenhagen G. The Scientific Section of the American Pharmaceutical Association. *Am J Pharm Ed.* 1953;17:342-50.
10. Higby G. *In Service to American Pharmacy: The Professional Life of William Procter, Jr.* Tuscaloosa, Ala: University of Alabama Press; 1992:78.

The Pharmaceutical Sciences in America, 1902-1952

*by John P. Swann**

T HE first half of the 20th century was a period of massive intellectual, institutional, and economic change in the pharmaceutical sciences. Investigations and doctoral training in the key basic biomedical sciences, such as physiology, biochemistry, and (to a lesser extent) pharmacology, had become institutionalized within a small group of leading American universities in the last quarter of the 19th century. This phenomenon had occurred many years earlier in Europe. Moreover, two European developments between 1890 and 1910, both of which were unassailable turning points in medical history, revealed the powerful potential of applying biomedical science to therapeutics. Beginning in 1890, advances in bacteriology and immunology provided a methodology for developing biologically derived cures for diphtheria and many other serious diseases. Twenty years later, Paul Ehrlich introduced a pharmaceutical, Salvarsan, designed to destroy the syphilis pathogen; this was the first chemotherapeutic agent. So, by the early years of the 20th century, science appeared to be on the brink of fashioning therapies that offered not just symptomatic relief but cure and prevention.

Academe was the principal institutional context for the fundamental advances that emerged in America, but some pharmaceutical companies quickly adopted scientific techniques for developing new drugs, beginning with antitoxins, sera, and vaccines in the 1890s. Being able to present itself as scientifically minded helped a firm project a progressive image to its clientele.[1] But investing in a scientific infrastructure also positioned a firm to compete in the race for new product development. In a sense, though, a firm wanting to engage in this race had no choice. The Biologics Control Act of 1902 mandated that any establishment wishing to produce immunologically derived treatments had to engage personnel who were scientifically equipped for the task.[2]

Few American pharmaceutical firms were willing to make the necessary

*John P. Swann, PhD, is Historian, Food and Drug Administration, Rockville, Md.

commitment to develop new biologicals or any other science-based medications. This became obvious during World War I, when the United States suffered shortages of key pharmaceuticals as a result of the nation's reliance on the German drug industry. The modern, research-based American pharmaceutical industry was born in the 1920s and 1930s as pharmaceutical firms developed their own research staffs and collaborated with pharmaceutical scientists in universities. Drug firms contributed directly to the advancement of knowledge by undergirding drug development. In addition, industry became a key source of fiscal support for many pharmaceutical scientists in universities long before the beginning of the federal government's systematic involvement.[3]

The government's support for drug research was relatively meager until the 1940s, but there were some exceptions. For example, the Interdepartmental Social Hygiene Board was created by the Chamberlain-Kahn Act of 1918 to coordinate research on venereal diseases. Its support for a collaborative arsenical research project involving pharmacologists at the University of Wisconsin, medicinal chemists at Northwestern University, and two psychiatric hospitals in Wisconsin in the 1920s led to the discovery of the value of tryparsamide in treating neurosyphilis. Also, after its establishment by Congress in 1937, the National Cancer Institute awarded 33 grants amounting to more than $200,000 in its first 2 years, including support for studies of cancer treatments.[4]

The 1940s witnessed a national commitment to drug and other biomedical research for wartime purposes. The Committee on Medical Research of the Office of Scientific Research and Development sponsored the research of more than 5,000 scientists and others through contracts valued at $25 million. Those contracts shifted to the National Institute of Health (as it was then known) at the end of the war. The World War II drug studies, which depended on hundreds of pharmacologists, medicinal chemists, and other biomedical scientists, are fairly well known. For example, attempts to prepare suitable antimalarial agents produced nearly two dozen that had some commercial success, such as amodiaquin. Although researchers were unable to prepare a commercially viable synthetic penicillin during the war, the chemical understanding of the drug that emerged from the program paved the way for the semisynthetic penicillins of the 1950s and after.[4, 5]

An analysis of the pharmaceutical sciences, such as pharmacology, medicinal chemistry, and pharmaceutics, during this period suggests that the different disciplines were at drastically different stages of development, particularly when one examines their growth in American schools of pharmacy. That pharmacy education overall moved slowly—even grudgingly—toward scientific rigor early in the 20th century complicated the adoption of some of the pharmaceutical sciences. A few pharmacy schools, such as those at the University of Michigan and University of Wisconsin, pioneered a science-based curriculum before the turn of the 20th century. Still, it was not until 1925 that a 3-year curriculum became mandatory for credentialed schools; a 4-year course became a requirement 7 years later. Graduate education in schools of pharmacy concomitantly lagged behind. By the early 1950s fewer than 20 schools offered doctoral training in the pharmaceutical sciences.[6]

The locus of practice notwithstanding, medicinal chemistry was probably on firmer footing in the first years of the 20th century than were the

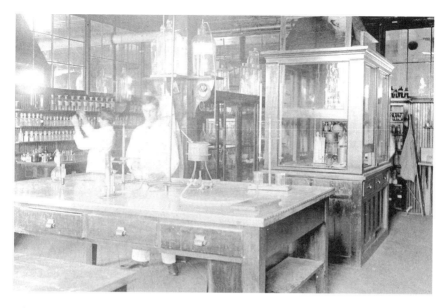

The progress in pharmaceutical sciences permitted pharmaceutical manu-facturers to enhance their drug product control procedures, as this photo of a pharmacological laboratory at Parke-Davis in 1900 shows.

other pharmaceutical sciences. This can be attributed to the solid institutional base of chemistry, generally, and organic and analytical chemistry, in particular. American successes in developing, reshaping, or gaining a greater understanding of pharmaceuticals can be seen throughout this half-century. A number of notable examples can be cited. Edward Calvin Kendall did pioneering work on both thyroxine and cortisone toward the beginning and the end of this half-century. The elaboration of anesthetics became a focal point of academic and industrial collaboration soon after World War I. Vitamins proliferated from the 1930s forward. More than 5,400 sulfonamide-related substances were prepared worldwide within a decade of the introduction of Prontosil in 1935 to improve its safety and effficacy (though the number of sulfas that made their way into medical practice was more on the order of dozens). John Sheehan developed a rational means for manipulating the molecular skeleton of penicillin to address the therapeutic problems associated with that wonder drug.[7-9]

Pharmacology became a vital element of pharmaceutical research in universities, the federal government, and industry early on in the half-century. For example, expertise in pharmacology enabled Parke-Davis to biologically standardize certain plant drugs in the 1890s, and it formed an integral part of the new drug programs at Lilly, Merck, Abbott, and other firms in the 1920s and 1930s. In the federal government, pharmacologists played an important role in the enforcement of biologics and food and drug laws and in a variety of research projects during the first half-century.

That discipline had a much stronger base in American medical schools than pharmacy schools. By 1910 there were several pharmacology chairs, a national association of pharmacologists, and a respected journal dedicated to pharmacology.[10] Most pharmacy schools were slow to embrace pharmacology for a variety of reasons, including the cost of providing the necessary laboratory space and the concern that teaching pharmacists the physiologic action and therapeutic uses of drugs would encourage them to counterprescribe. The traditional teaching of materia medica, with its emphasis on the pharmacognostic study of drugs, was a revered element of the curriculum, not easily usurped by a subject many pharmaceutical educators deemed more appropriately the province of physicians.[11]

A handful of schools were offering some instruction in pharmacology in 1908, when Rufus Lyman was appointed dean of the University of Nebraska School of Pharmacy. Lyman unswervingly championed pharmacology as a subject absolutely necessary in order to make it possible for pharmacists to "practice their profession intelligently."[12] By 1920 about half of the schools of pharmacy taught the subject—though the level of instruction varied. In 1927 the influential Charter Survey, representing pharmacy's educational, licensing, and retail interests, published *Basic Material for a Pharmaceutical Curriculum*. That monograph echoed Lyman's earlier sentiments. By the beginning of World War II, almost every pharmacy school offered laboratory-based instruction in pharmacology.[11]

Pharmaceutics, broadly conceived as the science of drug delivery, was founded on physicochemical principles derived from many different fields in several countries throughout the first half of the 20th century. For example, in the 1930s biophysicist Torsten Teorell in Sweden generated groundbreaking work on the kinetics of substances delivered through different routes of administration.[13, 14] However, by the end of this period schools of pharmacy and the pharmaceutical industry in the United States were emerging at the fore-

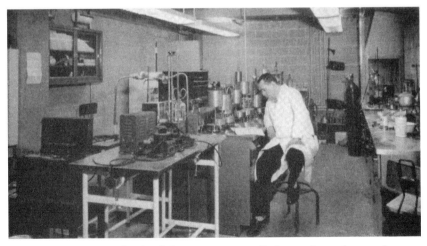

By the 1950s, more schools of pharmacy were offering grduate degrees in pharmaceutical sciences. This photograph shows an individual graduate laboratory at the University of Pittsburgh.

front of the field of pharmaceutics. Two developments are worth singling out. First, in 1947 the University of Wisconsin School of Pharmacy hired physical chemist Takeru Higuchi, whose leadership in physical pharmacy became legendary in that field. Second, in 1952 Smith Kline & French introduced the Spansule, a timed-release formulation that launched a widespread search for other applications of pharmaceutics to the design of dosage forms.[15, 16] Interest in dosage forms certainly was nothing new in the history of pharmacy, but this period gave rise to the development of a separate discipline that addressed the drug delivery system as a key component of therapeutics.

The pharmaceutical sciences underwent a metamorphosis from 1902 to 1952. Their advance was demonstrated by the expansion of the drug armamentarium itself, the tremendous growth of which was far too great to be characterized here. Different estates of science contributed, beginning with universities to be sure, but the pharmaceutical industry and the federal government also were very active participants. The last two were significant sources of research support during this period, with the government playing the larger role from World War II on.

By transitioning to a rigorous, biological science-based curriculum during this period, American pharmacy schools became another venue for the institutionalization of the pharmaceutical sciences. Pharmaceutical organizations contributed as well. The American Pharmaceutical Association had, almost since its founding, propagated a so-called query system that challenged members to carry out investigations addressing questions issued by the Association's executive committee.[17] The Scientific Section of APhA, which inherited the query system, became an important outlet for the presentation of results from scientific studies. From 1887 to 1953 more than 2,500 papers were presented before the Section.[18] These developments and others in the first five decades of the 20th century set the pharmaceutical sciences on a path toward revitalization and invigoration during the second half of the century.

This article originally appeared in *Journal of the American Pharmaceutical Association* 41, no. 6 (Nov/Dec 2001): 829-31.

References

1. Liebenau J. *Medical Science and Medical Industry: The Formation of the American Pharmaceutical Industry.* Baltimore, Md: Johns Hopkins University Press; 1987:57-78.
2. Kondratas RA Biologics Control Act of 1902. In: *The Early Years of Federal Food and Drug Control.* Madison, Wis: American Institute of the History of Pharmacy: 1982:8-27.
3. Swann JP. *Academic Scientists and the Pharmaceutical Industry: Cooperative Research in Twentieth-Century America.* Baltimore, Md: Johns Hopkins University Press; 1988.
4. Swann JP. Biomedical research and government support: the case of drug development. *Pharm Hist.* 1989;31:10-16.
5. Andrus EC Bronk DW, Carden GA Jr, et al., eds. *Advances in Military Medicine.* 2 vols. Boston, Mass: Little, Brown; 1948.
6. Sonnedecker G. *Kremers and Urdang's History of Pharmacy.* 4th ed. Philadelphia, Pa: Lippincott; 1976: 239-44.
7. Sneader W. *Drug Prototypes and Their Exploitation.* Chichester, Great Britain: John Wiley; 1996.

8. Goodman LS, Gilman A. *The Pharmacological Basis of Therapeutics*. 3rd ed. New York, NY: Macmillan, 1965: 1144.

9. Sheehan JC. *The Enchanted Ring: The Untold Story of Penicillin*. Cambridge, Mass: MIT Press; 1982.

10. Parascandola J. *The Development of American Pharmacology: John J. Abel and the Shaping of a Discipline*. Baltimore, Md: Johns Hopkins University Press; 1992.

11. Parascandola J, Swann J. Development of pharmacology in American schools of pharmacy. *Pharm Hist*. 1983 25:95-115.

12. Parascandola J, Swann J. Development of pharmacology in American schools of pharmacy. *Pharm Hist*. 1983; 25:101.

13. Wagner JG. The history of pharmacokinetics. *Drug Intell Clin Pharm*. 1977; 11 :747-8.

14. Wagner JG. The history of pharmacokinetics. *Pharmacol Ther*. 1981;12:537-62.

15. Swintosky JV. Personal adventures in biopharmaceutical research during the 1953-1984 years. *Drug Intell Clin Pharm*. 1985;19:265-76.

16. Helfand WH, Cowen DL. Evolution of pharmaceutical oral dosage forms. *Pharm Hist*. 1983;25:3-18.

17. Lynn EV. A century of research in pharmaceutical chemistry in the schools of pharmacy of the United States. *Am J Pharm Educ*. 1953;17:187-9.

18. Griffenhagen G. The Scientific Section of the American Pharmaceutical Association. *Am J Pharm Educ* 1953;17:342-50.

The Pharmaceutical Sciences in America, 1952-2002

by Edward G. Feldmann*

T HE past 50 years have brought enormous changes across the entire spectrum of human society, but nowhere have these new developments been more apparent than in the fields of science and technology. These scientific and technologic advances have had an especially profound impact on the fields of medicine and pharmacy.

In 1952 America experienced its most devastating annual epidemic of poliomyelitis; the entire nation was gripped with fear of this disease, commonly known as infantile paralysis. Thousands of victims died, and many survivors were consigned to living with braces, wheelchairs, or iron lungs.

Prior to the 1950s, the only preventive measure for polio—as for many other infectious diseases—was quarantine. But beginning in the late 1940s with the general availability of penicillin, an array of effective preventive and curative agents became available. Penicillin was followed by other antibiotics, as well as a host of effective biologic agents, including the Salk and Sabin polio vaccines. These "miracle" pharmaceuticals tamed or virtually eliminated many of the infections and contagious diseases then known.

This was the golden age of drug discovery—a span of 2 decades from the late 1940s through the late 1960s. Although many new drugs were subsequently developed, neither their number nor their clinical impact compared with the drugs that became available during that golden age. The chief thrust of new drug development during that fruitful period was the organic synthesis of new chemical entities often based on compounds isolated from natural products. However, by the end of the 20th century, the direction of new drug research had shifted dramatically.

Technology as a Major Catalyst

The human genome has been essentially decoded,[1] and, today, genetic manipulation is the underlying scientific approach to the newest therapeu-

*Now retired, Edward G. Feldmann, PhD, was the chief scientific staff officer at APhA for most of the period covered by this review with responsibility for all the Association's scientific activities described herein.

31

tic research.[2] Indeed, the present-day climate was concisely described in a recent article by pharmaceutical scientist Ronald T. Borchardt: "With the advent of genomics, proteomics, and bioinformatics, these [research-based pharmaceutical companies] now have access to an unprecedented abundance of potential therapeutic targets. With the emergence of combinatorial chemistry and innovative robotic-based technologies for conducting high throughput screening, these companies can also rapidly identify chemical leads that interact with these potential therapeutic targets. Using rational drug design strategies, promising leads can be rapidly optimized into high affinity ligands, referred to in the industry as new chemical entities."[3]

Although many factors might be cited as contributing to this monumental transition, two phenomena particularly stand out, namely, advances in technology and growth in size.

In Figure 1, a solitary scientist is shown in 1952 in what was at the time considered to be a well-equipped university research laboratory. Although well equipped, not a single electronic instrument can be seen in the laboratory for the simple reason that computers, pH meters, spectrophotometers, chromatographers, and other technical or electronic equipment either did not exist or were not yet generally available. In this laboratory computations were done with slide rules, not calculators.

"Chemistry without computers? Such was the world of 1976. . . . During the past 25 years, computers have revolutionized many areas of chemistry including the process of doing research,"[4] wrote a commentator tracing the 125-year history of the American Chemical Society. Today, test tubes, beakers, and flasks all the laboratory staples of the 1950s are almost completely gone, having been replaced by a vast array of instruments that allow scientists to work at submicro levels and to determine physical and chemical properties of a test sample that were undreamed of at mid-century.

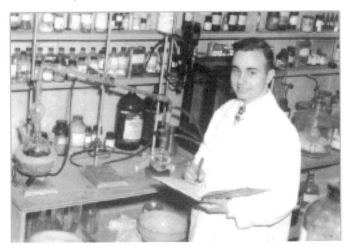

Figure 1. The author in his research laboratory at Loyola University (Chicago), April 1952. This organic chemistry laboratory—with an analytical balance, glassware with ground glass fittings, an electric heating mantle, and an electric stirring motor—was regarded as modern and well-equipped in its day. However, not a single electronic instrument is seen.

The New "Industrial Revolution"

In 1952 industrial research laboratories were miniscule in size by today's standards. Following World War II, the pharmaceutical industry largely consisted of such old-line firms as Eli Lilly, Upjohn, Squibb, Merrell, Abbott, Searle, and Parke-Davis, all of which had been founded by pharmacists or physicians and were still managed and operated by them or their family members. Those firms were all relatively small, often consisting of a single, factory-style building in which the research and control facilities shared space with all the other phases of drug product manufacturing and production. But with the industry's explosive growth, which began around 1950, the need for larger and more sophisticated research and quality control facilities and greater numbers of highly skilled personnel rapidly became apparent.

Although many industrial scientists and pharmaceutical firms contributed to the resultant growth, two pharmaceutical scientists—both with strong ties to pharmacy—stand out for their special leadership in this unprecedented expansion. Max Tischler at Merck and K.K. Chen at Eli Lilly were highly respected medicinal scientists as well as exceptionally able administrators.

For example, in 1960 Lilly was one of the first drug companies to devote an entire new building to its research endeavors. To mark the historic occasion of this building's dedication, the firm sponsored a special VIP seminar on the latest advances in quality control, to which it invited the quality control experts of that era. The industry's investment in research staff and facilities paid off handsomely; many new major drug discoveries were made and effective new dosage forms were developed.

The Influence of Academe

Although, to the public eye, great therapeutic strides were associated solely with the industry, such applied research discoveries and advances rested on the basic research conducted in academic institutions—principally, schools of pharmacy. Each branch of the pharmaceutical sciences underwent a major transition during the second half of the 20th century. For example, in 1950 pharmacognosy was presented essentially as the physical description of medicinal plant parts. But Varro Tyler and his colleagues revolutionized the field by emphasizing study of the important chemical constituents—notably alkaloids—of those plant materials. Similarly, pharmaceutical analysis had mainly consisted of "wet chemistry," in which visual observation of color changes, precipitate formation, and other crude procedures were employed. Comparison of the *United States Pharmacopeia/National Formulary* (USP/NF) monographs of 1950 with those in the 2000 compendia reveal differences as dramatic as comparing a 1950 Piper Cub airplane with today's Space Shuttle.

Although all branches of the pharmaceutical sciences experienced similar sea changes, changes in dosage form design, development, and manufacture were arguably the most dramatic. In the early 1950s a young physical chemist on the faculty of the University of Wisconsin School of Pharmacy, Takeru Higuchi, began to research the application of physical chemistry principles to drug dosage forms, and the new science of physical pharmacy was conceived. Over the next 3 decades Higuchi's influence proved to be enormous as he trained a large cadre of graduate students who subsequently disseminated this new concept throughout both academe and industry.

This marriage of pharmacy and physical chemistry gave rise to totally new dosage forms, such as timed-release and delayed-release products, as well as new drug delivery systems, such as transdermal patches and osmotic pumps. It also resulted in the recognition of the importance and, therefore, the study of drug transport, pharmacokinetics, and the fundamental concepts of drug absorption, distribution, metabolism, and excretion.

Playing an important complementary role were the USP, NF, and the U.S. Food and Drug Administration. These standard-setting and standard-enforcing agencies sought to assure the quality, reliability, and uniformity of pharmaceuticals in the marketplace. Bioavailability surfaced as a key property of commercial drug dosage forms. The profitability of drug firms, the financial viability of government social programs, and similar crucial economic consequences revolved around generic equivalency, and the latter rested on determinations of comparable levels of bioavailability. In this regard, the official compendia and their modest laboratory facility (the Drug Standards Laboratory) provided needed leadership and impetus for research on associated testing methodology.

APhA as Patron of the Sciences

The role, influence, and impact of APhA in helping to foster the unimaginable changes and progress of the pharmaceutical sciences during the past 50 years cannot be overstated. Two previous articles in this series[5,6] clearly traced the nurturing role the Association played during its first century. This proactive, positive influence was even greater during the past half-century. Specifically, APhA fostered the pharmaceutical sciences by:

•Providing a home base for its science-oriented members. From 1887 until 1965, an APhA organizational unit titled the Scientific Section offered a primary forum for the presentation of research reports at APhA Annual Meetings. Then, in 1966, APhA underwent a major reorganization that included the establishment of the Academy of Pharmaceutical Sciences with greatly expanded member services and a full-time staff. Subsequently, in 1986, out of this unit sprang the independent American Association of Pharmaceutical Scientists.

•Providing outlets for the publication of original scientific research as well as comprehensive monographs on scientific subjects. Most prominent in this regard is the *Journal of Pharmaceutical Sciences*, now in its 91st year as the "grand-daddy" of pharmacy research periodicals. This premier journal evolved through several name changes, with the current title selected in 1961 to convey its expanded mission to serve the entire community of pharmaceutical scientists and not just APhA members. In 1961 the concept of "pharmaceutical sciences" was still in its infancy.

•Providing science-based mechanisms to ensure drug quality and effectiveness.

This role was filled by APhA's sponsorship of the NF from 1888 until it was merged with the USP in 1975, including the operation of the Drug Standards Laboratory in the APhA Headquarters building.

• Providing incentives, encouragement, and recognition to individual pharmaceutical scientists. APhA established the first awards and honors to be bestowed in recognition of noteworthy pharmaceutical scientific contributions. In the early 1960s the Association greatly expanded its awards program to cover all the individual sciences. It also broke new ground in providing opportunities for women in the science of pharmacy; notably, in the late 1960s, APhA was the first organization to appoint a woman, Mary Hudson Ferguson, PhD, as editor of its research journal, and, in the mid-1980s, Lucinda Maine, PhD, became the Association's principal science staff officer.

Conclusion

The pharmaceutical sciences occupy a crucial place in the evolution of American pharmacy in general and of APhA in particular. This is as it should be, since the pharmaceutical sciences provide the foundation and underpinning for the current practice of pharmacy as well as the expanded roles pharmacy practitioners are expected to fill now or in the near future: drug product selection, over-the-counter drug advice and recommendations, therapeutic counseling, drug interaction monitoring and detection, and full partnership with physicians and other health care practitioners in determining optimal and individualized patient therapy. Sir Isaac Newton is reported to have said, "If I have seen further . . . it is by standing upon the shoulders of giants." To paraphrase this quote, if today's pharmacists are more effective and meaningful health care practitioners, it is because they stand firmly on a solid base of the pharmaceutical sciences.

This article originally appeared in *Journal of the American Pharmaceutical Association*, 42, no. 6 (Nov/Dec 2002): 828-30.

References

1. Emmett A. The human genome. *The Scientist*. July 24, 2000:1.
2. Roth RI, Fleischer NM. Gene therapy: applications to pharmacy practice. *J Am Pharm Assoc*. 2002;42:692-8.
3. Borchardt RT. Integrating drug discovery and development. *The Scientist*. March 5, 2001:43.
4. Venere E. 125th Anniversary focus. *Chemistry*. Summer 2001;14.
5. Parascandola J. The pharmaceutical sciences in America, 1852–1902. *J Am Pharm Assoc*. 2000;40:733–5.
6. Swann JP. The pharmaceutical sciences in America, 1902–1952. *J Am Pharm Assoc*. 2001;41:829–31.

American Pharmaceutical Education, 1852-1902

by Robert A. Buerki*

In 1854 a Committee on Education appointed by the newly formed American Pharmaceutical Association (APhA) complained that the country had been

deluged with incompetent drug clerks [employee pharmacists], whose claim to the important position they hold or apply for is based on a year or two's service in the shop, perhaps under conditions illy calculated to increase their knowledge. These clerks in turn become principals, and have the direction of others-alas! for the progeny that some of them bring forth, as ignorance multiplied by ignorance will produce neither knowledge nor skill.

Significantly, the committee, led by Philadelphia's William Procter, Jr., and Edward Parrish, did not expect drug clerks or even apprentices to study pharmacy formally. It merely admonished them read the pharmaceutical literature "regularly and understandingly" and assist their reading "by experiment and observation" when necessary.[1]

Procter and Parrish had good reason to be concerned. Unlike physicians, who created medical schools and societies and agitated for protective legislation as early as the 1760s, nineteenth-century American apothecaries clung to an informal system of apprenticeship that lacked the standards that strong English guilds had once given it. Until 1865, formal instruction in the practice of pharmacy was given in a medical school in New Orleans and in five independent schools operated by pharmacists through local associations called "colleges of pharmacy."[a,2] In Philadelphia (1821), New York (1829), Baltimore (1841), Chicago (1859), and St. Louis (1865), these schools sought to supplement the practical information gathered by apprentices during

---

*Robert A. Buerki, PhD, is professor of pharmacy practice and administration, College of Pharmacy, The Ohio State University, Columbus.

[a]A pharmacy curriculum established in 1838 within the Medical College of Louisiana at New Orleans and, after 1847, as part of the University of Louisiana (now Tulane University) claims historical priority in instruction, but not as a separately constituted school or college of pharmacy. See Reference 2.

37

their in-service training, organizing the scattered fragments into a systematic whole. Physicians and, later, master pharmacists provided instruction in the form of lectures two or three evenings a week during the winter months. There were no requirements for admission, save perhaps apprenticeship with some preceptor; apprentices would attend the same lectures twice in successive winters or possibly more often; there was little laboratory instruction available. To graduate, apprentices had to pass an examination given by the lecturers and an examining committee of the college and show proof of a satisfactory apprenticeship of 4 years, which included "attendance upon lectures." The number of apprentices attending lectures in these schools before the Civil War was small, and the number who graduated was still smaller: of the 11,031 apothecaries and druggists in the United States in 1860, only 514 had graduated from a pharmacy course, most from the school in Philadelphia.[3,4]

After the Civil War, pharmacy schools were formed in one of four ways: privately by groups of pharmacists organized only for that purpose; as parts of private or denominational universities and colleges; as divisions of medical colleges; or, most importantly, as parts of state universities. The Morrill Land Grant Act (1862) underscored the belief that higher education should be made available to broader segments of the American public. Funded by sales of lands in the western territories, states were to establish public universities that would focus on education in the applied sciences, perform broad public service, and engage in activities designed to serve the people. To the struggling health professions in mid-nineteenth-century America, the act brought hope for stability and increased recognition; to the increasingly cramped and limited system of American pharmaceutical education, the effect of the Morrill Act was no less than profound.

The first state-supported institution to produce graduates in pharmacy was the Medical College of the State of South Carolina (1867), but the real revolution began in 1868 at the University of Michigan, with neither the support of the pharmacists in the state nor the legitimizing influence of a state pharmacy practice act. In a bold innovation, physician-chemist Albert B. Prescott introduced a 2-year course of instruction that included ample labo-

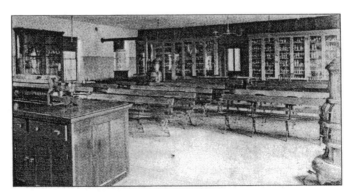

The Pharmaceutical Lecture Room at the University of Wisconsin in Madison soon after the school was established in 1883.

ratory work in pharmaceutical chemistry, microscopic botany, and pharmacy, but required no apprenticeship as a prerequisite to graduation. Prescott's rejection of the time-honored notion that academic instruction should merely round off an extended apprenticeship, coupled with the profession's fear of encroaching "state control" of education, quickly made him an unpopular figure in pharmaceutical circles. A "Conference of Schools of Pharmacy" organized by association-based schools in 1870 declared that diplomas should not be recognized unless they were based on "four years' practical service in a dispensing shop."[5,6] Prescott explained the advantages of a scientific education for pharmacists before the APhA meeting the following year, but his school was refused recognition as a college of pharmacy because it did not ensure the "proper practical training" to its graduates; moreover, only five states had adopted legislation defining the practice of pharmacy and limiting that practice to qualified practitioners. Commitment to the educational ideology of the association-based schools and insistence on developing pharmaceutical education independently from the medical profession would continue to hamper educational progress for another decade. The conference quietly expired in 1884, because the delegates lacked authority to make decisions for their colleges. Its ambitions never went beyond that of a sounding board and advisory discussion group, Sonnedecker has noted, and its mechanism protected against unwelcome or inconvenient innovations.[7,8]

In 1883 the second state-supported school of pharmacy was founded at the University of Wisconsin at the request of the state pharmaceutical association and on the heels of a new state pharmacy practice act. Unlike Prescott, pharmacist-scientist Frederick B. Power made practical experience a requirement for a diploma, although not a prerequisite for admission. Since 1871, 11 private and practitioner-controlled proprietary schools had been founded, but only 5 survived by later affiliating with a private or public university. During this same period, pharmacists in 31 states had formed state pharmaceutical associations; these associations, in turn, had stimulated the passage of 15

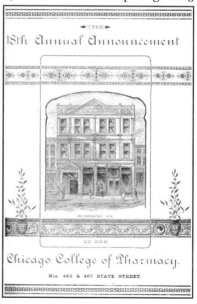

In 1884-1885, the Chicago College of Pharmacy offered the Graduate in Pharmacy (PhG) degree for a 2-year course, with "practical instruction in pharmaceutical laboratory work" under the direction of Oscar Oldberg.

new state pharmacy practice acts. In 1887 a reorganized APhA established four sections to debate scientific issues, commercial interests, pharmaceutical education, and legislation. A merged Section on Education and Legislation (1890) collected and published data and provided a much-needed forum for discussion on educational issues and emerging legislation, but when Chicago's Carl S. N. Hallberg offered a resolution to require "theoretical education" in a school or college of pharmacy as a prerequisite for examination and registration as a pharmacist "in the nearest possible future" at the 1892 meeting, the proposal was subjected to a withering barrage of criticism and withdrawn.[9,10] Nevertheless, the continuing debates within the Section would spark the creation of the American Conference of Pharmaceutical Faculties in 1900, ushering in a new era of progress in pharmaceutical education.

The new pharmacy practice laws of the 1880s were not retroactive, but merely recognized and registered those pharmacists in practice at the time without an examination. For those entering the profession, the new laws required only proof of some apprenticeship and enough knowledge to pass the examination. Apprentices were often referred to the standard textbooks of the day, the *United States Dispensatory*, or Joseph P. Remington's *The Practice of Pharmacy*. Another type of preparation, restricted to mastering questions commonly asked in the examination, promised easier success. Correspondence courses through pharmaceutical journals flourished, typified by the "National Institute of Pharmacy," launched in 1885 by Hallberg, publisher of *The Western Druggist* and professor at the Chicago College of Pharmacy, and "The Era Course of Pharmacy," introduced in 1897 by Ohio's James H. Beal, dean of the Scio College Department of Pharmacy, which featured the nation's most outstanding pharmaceutical scientists and educators as authors. Apprentices not willing to endure the discipline set by the burgeoning correspondence courses sought less formidable study aids, typified by *A Course of Home Study for Pharmacists*, first published in 1891 by Oscar Oldberg, dean of the Illinois College of Pharmacy at Northwestern University. While Oldberg's ambitious home study book received high praise, its less respectable counterpart, the "quiz-compend," collections of questions commonly asked in the state board examinations, received strong condemnation from pharmaceutical educators and editors alike. Nevertheless, such slender volumes as Francis E. Stewart's *A Compend of Pharmacy*, which first appeared in 1886, enjoyed enormous popularity for more than four decades.[11]

The stability of the state colleges and universities would prove their merit: of the 19 state-sponsored schools and colleges of pharmacy founded between 1884 and 1902, only 3 would fail. In stark contrast, of the 38 private, proprietary, association-based, or medical school-based schools and colleges of pharmacy founded during this period, only 3 survived intact, 9 others merging or affiliating with public or private universities.[12] Moreover, in 1892, Edward Kremers introduced the first 4-year baccalaureate degree in pharmacy at the University of Wisconsin, placing the study of pharmacy on a par with other academic majors. The emerging aura of professionalism fostered a new spirit of cooperation among former rival factions: APhA advocated an increased dependence on diplomas and licenses to meet new professional challenges; schools and boards of pharmacy now worked together on apprenticeships, board examinations, and course content. As boards imposed practical experience requirements for licensure, they released schools and colleges of pharmacy from enforcing similar experience for graduation. While the old-line association schools continued to cling to the apprenticeship model for pharmaceutical education, the newer university-based schools and colleges of pharmacy pressed for full academic recognition as an applied scientific discipline. Resolution of these and other educational issues would wait upon an invigorated professional leadership within pharmacy during the first decades of the new century.

This article originally appeared in *Journal of the American Pharmaceutical Association*, 40, no. 4 (July /Aug 2000): 458-60.

References

1. Procter W Jr, Parrish E, Stewart D, Meakim J. Report of the Committee on Education: Address to the Pharmaceutists of the United States. *Proc Am Pharm Assoc.* 1854(3):14-5,20.
2. Dyer JP. *Tulane: The Biography of a University, 1834-1965.* New York, NY: Harper & Row; 1966:21,70n,134.
3. Taylor H. Schools and Colleges of Pharmacy. *Pharmaceutical Era.* 1912;45(5):336.
4. Sonnedecker GA. American Pharmaceutical Education Before 1900 [dissertation]. Madison, WI: University of Wisconsin; 1952:52 n. 17.
5. Wright Jr W. Minutes of the Convention of Delegates from Colleges and Societies of Pharmacy, Held in Baltimore on the 14th and 15th of September, Relative to Pharmaceutical Education. *Am J Pharm.* 1870;42(6):504.
6. Sonnedecker GA. The Conference of Schools of Pharmacy-A Period of Frustration. *Am J Pharm Educ.* 1954;18:400-1.
7. Markoe GFH, Doliber T, Bedford PW, et al. Report of the Committee on the Credentials of the Delegate from the University of Michigan. *Proc Am Pharm Assoc.* 1871;19:47.
8. Prescott AB. Pharmaceutical Education. *Proc Am Pharm Assoc.* 1871;19:425-9.
9. Rapelye CA. Section on Pharmaceutical Education and Legislation: Second Session-Monday Afternoon, July 18. *Proc Am Pharm Assoc.* 1892;40:333.
10. Section on Pharmaceutical Education and Legislation: Second Session-Monday Afternoon, July 18. Discussion. *Proc Am Pharm Assoc.* 1892;40:333-8.
11. Buerki RA. Historical Perspective. In: *Continuing Education in Pharmacy.* Arndt JR, Coons SJ. Alexandria, Va: American Association of Colleges of Pharmacy; 1987:11-2.
12. Sonnedecker GA. *Kremers and Urdang's History of Pharmacy*, 4th ed. Philadelphia, Pa: J.B. Lippincott Co; 1976:384-5.

American Pharmaceutical Education, 1902-1952

by Robert A. Buerki*

I̶ₙ a keynote address read before the Golden Jubilee Meeting of the American Pharmaceutical Association (APhA) in Philadelphia in 1902, the influential German pharmacist Frederick Hoffmann drew attention to "the prevailing ill-advised tendency toward the excessive multiplication of all grades and all kinds of schools and institutions of pharmacy." Warming to his topic, Hoffmann continued:

There remains cause for apprehension as to maintaining unimpaired the established standards and the integrity of pharmaceutical education. The most serious drawback from which pharmaceutical education in our country has always suffered is the unrestricted low standard of the preliminary education of most men entering the drug trade.[1]

At that same meeting, APhA President Henry M. Whelpley rekindled the debate over the primacy of apprenticeship, which had divided pharmacy educators and practitioners for nearly half a century. "We not permit the newcomers to obscure the real foundation of the education of those who are to be successors as the compounders and dispensers of medicines," Whelpley remarked. "The qualifications for entering college should pertain to the lifework of the matriculant as well as meet the demands of the college course."[2]

Establishing educational criteria would prove challenging. At the turn of the century, the typical course of study in pharmacy covered 2 years, but 3- and 4-year courses were available. The school year varied across institutions from 23 to 42 weeks; most colleges were run as day schools, but evening sessions were not uncommon. Admission requirements ranged from no educational requirements at all to high school graduation, with the majority of colleges requiring only the completion of an elementary or grammar school education. Most colleges conferred the graduate in pharmacy (PhG) degree, but others conferred the pharmaceutical chemist (PhC) degree, the BS, or the

---

*Robert A. Buerki, PhD, is professor of pharmacy practice and administration, College of Pharmacy, The Ohio State University, Columbus, OH.

43

PharmD. Some colleges required specified amounts of practical experience for one or more of their degrees; others imposed no such requirements.[3,4]

The American Conference of Pharmaceutical Faculties (ACPF), organized in 1900, struggled to bring some order to the curricular chaos that reigned in the United States, but by 1903 ACPF could only agree that its 23 member institutions should have been "in continuous operation in America" for at least 5 years, their applicants be at least 17 years of age and have completed a "common school education, entitling the student to enter high school," and their graduates complete not less than 500 hours of lectures and recitations and 600 hours of laboratory work over a period of not less than 40 weeks, none of which was to be offered in absentia.[5,6] The modest requirements did not apply to the other 57 schools and colleges of pharmacy that were not members of the Conference.

The movement to require graduation from a school or college of pharmacy as a condition for sitting for a state board of pharmacy examination began at the 1891 meeting of the APhA Section on Education and Legislation, but was soundly defeated by board members who felt that the profession was not ready to take such an advanced step.[7] What could not be accomplished at the national level was pursued by state pharmaceutical associations in the form of so-called "prerequisite legislation." In 1904 the New York State Pharmaceutical Association pushed a compromise bill through its state legislature requiring applicants for licensure to be 21 years of age, have 4 years of practical experience, and pass an entrance examination covering 12 specific high school credits. Institutions were required to register with the Board of Regents, teach a 2-year course, and maintain a "proper pharmacy standard."[8] A less stringent measure, requiring only 4 years of practical experience and graduation from "some reputable and properly chartered college of pharmacy," was adopted by the Pennsylvania legislature the following year.[9]

While Pennsylvania's state board of pharmacy—and others—simply recognized membership in the ACPF as sufficient to meet the standards of their prerequisite laws, the New York legislation presented pharmaceutical education with a formidable challenge. The law specified that approved institutions maintain "a proper pharmacy standard," but failed to define such a standard.[10] At first, a "Committee of Three" New York representatives was appointed to set the standard, but it soon became apparent that such an activity could have greater value if it had a national scope. In 1906 the New York committee invited the National Association of Boards of Pharmacy (NABP) and ACPF to elect representatives to a National Syllabus Committee.[11] The enlarged committee considered all subjects found in the curriculums of the nation's schools and colleges of pharmacy, as well as the examinations of the state boards of pharmacy over the next several years, and narrowed them down to an outline for a 2-year course of study. Its findings were published in February 1910 as *The Pharmaceutical Syllabus*.[12]

ACPF, NABP, and APhA amended their bylaws to make provision for permanent representation on a new National Syllabus Committee, making the Syllabus an integral part of the structure of American pharmacy. By 1913, 62 of the 83 schools and colleges of pharmacy in the United States had formally adopted the Syllabus; a second edition was published in 1913, a third in 1922, and a fourth in 1932.[13]

During this period, the Syllabus provided a much-needed stabilizing

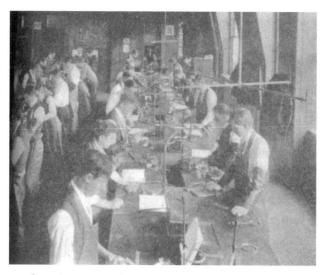

Pharmacy students in 1911 receive instruction in compounding at the University of Illinois School of Pharmacy.

influence on the interface between the requirements for pharmacy practice and the requirements of a standardized curriculum that both ACPF and non-ACPF schools could support, prompting the passage of a flurry of prerequisite legislation, particularly after 1915.[14] By 1925, 27 states had prerequisite laws on their books and others were considering the issue.[14] By 1932 the American Association of Colleges of Pharmacy (AACP), which subsumed ACPF in 1925, had achieved remarkable progress. During its first 3 decades, it had secured high school graduation as an entrance requirement for member institutions (1925) and approved a 4-year baccalaureate pharmacy program (1928), to become effective in 1932. That same year, the American Council on Pharmaceutical Education (ACPE) was created to accredit the new programs, replacing the cumbersome system of "official visits" the AACP had put in place to monitor the educational standards of its member institutions.[13,15]

As the Great Depression settled in, enrollment in America's schools and colleges of pharmacy plummeted to only 1,780 students in 1932,[16] and then rebounded, reassuring pharmacy educators that the science-based baccalaureate program they had struggled so long to attain had been justified, at least by the measure of increased enrollment.[17] World War II brought another precipitous drop in enrollment as pharmacy students were refused special deferments and whisked into the Armed Services through the draft. America's schools and colleges of pharmacy responded by accelerating and compressing their 4-year programs to 32 or even 24 months of year-round study. During these same years, *The Pharmaceutical Syllabus*, which had become more rigid and less responsive to change with each successive edition, lost favor among pharmacy educators, particularly when ACPE considered making its standards obligatory. By August 1946 all three sponsoring associations had withdrawn their support of the Syllabus.[18]

In the intervening years, pharmaceutical science and technology had exploded, leading some pharmacy educators and leaders to conclude that the 4-year curriculum was inadequate; others pointed to the paucity of the general education portion of the curriculum and the difficulty of attracting talented students directly from high school. In 1946 the American Council on Education, supported by grants from the American Foundation for Pharmaceutical Education, launched The Pharmaceutical Survey, still the most comprehensive and influential survey on American pharmacy practice and education ever conducted. In 1948 a poll of pharmacy deans revealed an even split between retaining the 4-year program and extending the pharmacy curriculum. That same year, the Committee on The Pharmaceutical Survey released its preliminary findings urging AACP and ACPE to "continue their efforts for the constructive betterment" of the 4-year program and establish an optional "program of education and training leading to the professional degree of Doctor of Pharmacy." Five-year baccalaureate programs, pioneered by Ohio State University in 1948, were dismissed by the Committee as leaving "much to be desired."[19,20]

Over the next 4 years, the preliminary findings of The Pharmaceutical Survey were hotly debated in pharmacy circles. Despite its initial enthusiasm, AACP's discussions quickly became mired in debates over the relative merits of 4-, 5-, and 6-year educational programs and in parliamentary maneuvering. Both APhA and the National Association of Retail Druggists publicly questioned the need for a 6-year program,[15] prompting the Committee on The Pharmaceutical Survey to soften its recommendations: only "adequately staffed and financed, and favorably located" institutions were urged to develop 6-year doctoral programs; 4-year programs would provide the "minimum mandatory training necessary for the practice of pharmacy."[21] In 1951 AACP delegates narrowly defeated a proposal that would have required member colleges to offer only a 5-year program after July 1, 1956.[15] At the time, 13 institutions were offering longer baccalaureate programs; the University of Southern California offered the 6-year PharmD as its only degree, beginning in 1950.[22]

A booming postwar economy had stimulated unprecedented changes in pharmacy practice, showing educators that they could no longer predict future trends with any confidence. The progressive, goal-oriented curricular development which had characterized the first 4 decades of the new century had given way to a decade of introspection and indecision. A practitioner-based "clinical pharmacy" movement and a new, patient-centered practice philosophy would set the tone for curricular development during the next 50 years.

This article originally appeared in *Journal of the American Pharmaceutical Association*, 41, no.4 (July/Aug 2001): 519-21.

References

1. Hoffmann F. A retrospect of the development of American pharmacy and the American Pharmaceutical Association. *Proc Am Pharm Assoc*. 1902;50:139.
2. Whelpley HM. The American Pharmaceutical Association in 1902. *Proc Am Pharm Assoc*. 1902;50:10.
3. U.S. Bureau of Education. Table 13. Statistics of schools of pharmacy for the year 1899-1900. *Report of the Commissioner of Education for the Year 1899-1900*. Vol. 2. Washington, DC: Government Printing Office; 1901:2008-11

4. Taylor HL. *Professional Education in the United States: Pharmacy*. Albany, NY: University of the State of New York; 1900:963-98.
5. Whelpley HM. Report of the Executive Committee. *Proc Am Conf Pharm Faculties*. 1904;5:34.
6. Qualifications for admission to and membership in the American Conference of Pharmaceutical Faculties. *Proc Am Conf Pharm Faculties*. 1904;5:35.
7. Remington JP. The recognition of college diplomas by state pharmacy laws. *Proc Am Pharm Assoc*. 1891;39:195-98, 198-204
8. Passage of the prerequisite bill. *Am Drug Pharm Rec*. 1904;44(8):247.
9. Remington JP. The recognition of the college diploma. *Am J Pharm*. 1905;77(4):183-5.
10. Mason HB. Chairman's address. *Proc Am Pharm Assoc*. 1905;53:105-6.
11. Taylor HL. Report of the National Syllabus Committee. *Proc Am Conf Pharm Faculties*. 1907;8:29.
12. Preface. *The Pharmaceutical Syllabus*. 1st ed. Albany, NY: New York State Board of Pharmacy; 1910:12-16.
13. Blauch LE, Webster GL. *The Pharmaceutical Curriculum*. Washington, DC: American Council on Education; 1952:21,15-6.
14. Day WB. Report of the Committee on Distribution of Information Concerning Prerequisite Legislation. *Proc Am Assoc Coll Pharm*. 1925;26:39-40.
15. Buerki RA. In search of excellence: the first century of the American Association of Colleges of Pharmacy. *Am J Pharm Educ*. 1999;63(fall suppl):55-9,117-20.
16. Jordan CB. Report of the Executive Committee. *Proc Am Assoc Coll Pharm*. 1933;34:42.
17. Little E. Registration in association colleges during the past fifteen years. *J Am Pharm Assoc (Pract Pharm Ed)*. 1940;10:366-67.
18. Mrtek RG. Pharmaceutical education in these United States: an interpretive historical essay of the twentieth century. *Am J Pharm Educ*. 1976;40:351-2.
19. Blauch LE The survey has looked at the pharmaceutical curriculum. *Am J Pharm Educ*. 1948;12:691-92.
20. Section X. *The pharmaceutical curriculum. Findings and Recommendations of the Pharmaceutical Survey, 1948*. Washington, DC: American Council on Education; 1948:45.
21. Elliott EC. Part XI. The findings and recommendations: section 10. The pharmaceutical curriculum. *The General Report of the Pharmaceutical Survey, 1946-49*. Washington, DC: American Council on Education; 1950:229-30.
22. Burt JB. Report of the Executive Committee, The American Association of Colleges of Pharmacy, Association Year 1951-52. *Am J Pharm Educ* . 1952;16:573-74.

American Pharmaceutical Education, 1952-2002

*By Robert A. Buerki**

"P HARMACY is the only member of the healing arts whose educational system is not required to be based on preprofessional education at the college level," President-Elect Richard Q. Richards told listeners at the Centennial Convention of the American Pharmaceutical Association (APhA) in Philadelphia in 1952. "We should soon be revising our program to permit a full year of specialization and this cannot be accomplished in three years of professional study."[1] Louis J. Fischl, chairman of the House of Delegates, in his address to the Convention, agreed: "There is no longer any doubt in my mind for the necessity of a five-year curriculum, including one year of pre-pharmacy."[2]

These clarion calls for action underscored recommendations published earlier that year in Lloyd E. Blauch and George L. Webster's *The Pharmaceutical Curriculum.*[3] Undertaken as an important component of the Pharmaceutical Survey of 1946-1948 but published under the auspices of the American Council on Education, this controversial little red book survived an "inquisition for radicalism" prompted by its authors' faint praise for 4-year pharmacy programs and their vision of pharmacy curricula "based on prior college education (five- and six-year plans)." In 1976 Robert G. Mrtek characterized *The Pharmaceutical Curriculum* as "the single most influential force on curriculum construction for at least two decades after its appearance."[4] In studied contrast, delegates to the 1952 meeting of the American Association of Colleges of Pharmacy (AACP) continued to debate a proposal that would have required member colleges to offer only a 5-year program. While pharmaceutical education had led practice during the preceding 50 years, the cold war mentality that had gripped the nation seemed to extend its grasp to pharmacy educators, creating a mind set that would stultify true educational reform for the next 4 decades.

By 1953, pressures to develop a solid prepharmacy curriculum had become irresistible. "With all the drugs that must be studied today it is almost

---

*Robert A. Buerki, PhD, is professor of pharmacy practice and administration, College of Pharmacy, Ohio State University, Columbus, OH.

impossible to cram it into four years and still obtain a well-rounded education," Madeline Oxford Holland, editor of the *American Professional Pharmacist*, complained. "We believe that the pharmacist needs more of the cul-
tural subjects as well as the technical courses which are necessary for him to
practice his profession."[5] APhA's secretary, the redoubtable Robert P. Fischelis, agreed: "No responsible educator or member of our profession has advocated an increase in the length of the professional course in pharmacy," he
stormed. "Let us recognize that adequate preparation for the study of pharmacy requires more than a four-year high school course, as twenty percent of
our accredited colleges have already done."[6]

At its 1953 annual meeting, the National Association of Boards of Pharmacy (NABP) passed a resolution favoring the adoption of the 5-year program
as the "minimum requirement for graduation";[7] APhA resolutions urged the
adoption of a "minimum combined program of preprofessional and professional education of at least five years," and further urged AACP and NABP to
"make such a program mandatory without delay."[8] Other endorsements came
from the American College of Apothecaries (ACA), the American Society of
Hospital Pharmacists, and the National Council of State Association Secretaries.[9] Despite strong opposition from trade associations, AACP approved a
proposal in 1954 to require "completion of not less than five full academic
years of training" for a degree in pharmacy "on and after April 1, 1965,"[10]
ending a debate over preliminary education that had consumed pharmacy
educators since 1941.[11]

Over the next 3 decades, the American practice of pharmacy would be
transformed in ways scarcely comprehensible to pharmacists of earlier gen-
erations. Between 1948 and 1960, the number of prescriptions dispensed
increased by nearly 70%, accounting for nearly a 4-fold increase in prescription dollar volume; by the end of the 1960s, these figures would double
again, reflecting physicians' increased use of more effective, single-ingredient
therapeutic agents, the aggressive promotion of brand-name drugs by pharmaceutical manufacturers, and the growth of the "third party payment" phenomenon. Indeed, by 1974, some third party was paying at least part of the
cost of one out of every four prescriptions dispensed.[12-14]

The consumerism movement of the early 1970s focused the American
public's attention on professional accountability, which resulted in mandated continued professional education and enhance standards of practice,
which were debated extensively and finally set down on paper in 1979. To
some educators, the rapid growth in the use of generic drug products and
the subsequent repeal of antisubstitution laws signaled the need for pharmacists to expand their role in advising physicians about drug product selection,
particularly in the institutional setting, where pharmacists participated in the
deliberations of pharmacy and therapeutics committees.

In the community setting, computerized patient record systems transformed the pharmacist's informational function from merely collecting,
retrieving, and transmitting data to interpreting clinically significant drug
interactions, a role for which many pharmacists were ill-prepared. At the
same time, a new breed of clinical pharmacists argued persuasively that
professional redemption lay in a radical shift from a product-oriented to
a patient-oriented practice, one that emphasized patient counseling and a
revolutionary change in practice philosophy crystallized by the term "phar-

maceutical care."[15-17]

The initial response to this sea change in professional practice by schools and colleges of pharmacy was predictable. Pharmacy faculties, dominated by pharmaceutical scientists, saw one path to the salvation of the pharmacy curriculum—Add more pharmaceutical science courses. Instructors of pharmacology, biochemistry, natural products chemistry, and pharmaceutics vied for space in crowded 5-year pharmacy curricula already stretched to the breaking point with general education electives.

Reactions from within and outside the profession were predictable as well. In an address before APhA's 1964 Annual Meeting, physician Henry T. Clark, Jr., charged that schools and colleges of pharmacy had neither "responded well" to the call for leadership during the preceding 2 decades of social and scientific change nor "provided guidelines for the growth of the profession."[18] That same year, ACA executive secretary Robert E. Abrams declared that education for the science of pharmacy had so outstripped education for the profession of pharmacy that the development of good practitioners was being neglected.[19] Even the University of California-San Francisco's dean Jere E. Goyan could complain that the educational system had turned out "a generation of pharmacists who knew the chemical structures of phenobarbital and procaine, including several pathways to their synthesis, and other arcane knowledge for which, to put it politely, they found little use."[20]

Pharmacy educators reacted cautiously to these criticisms, adding externship experiences mandated by the American Council on Pharmaceutical Education (ACPE) and trotting out courses in anatomy, physiology, pathophysiology, and biopharmaceutics to replace offerings in analytical chemistry, pharmacognosy, and industrial pharmacy, but they stopped short of developing curricula firmly grounded in the principles of clinical pharmacy. During the early 1970s, in exchange for generous federal capitation grants requiring development of a clinical component in their curricula, America's schools and colleges of pharmacy added literally hundreds of full- and part-time clinical instructors to their science-based faculties. The resulting academic atmosphere was often tense, or even hostile, as tenure-track faculty struggled to maintain control over curricular decisions and rapidly diminishing resources for research and graduate education.[21] By the late 1970s, however, this opposition began to wane as regular faculty realized that they had little to fear from their clinical brethren; both were now working toward a common goal—to improve the quality of pharmaceutical education.

These same years saw the publication of a number of national studies of pharmacy practice containing recommendations that would have a profound effect on pharmaceutical education. In *Pharmacists for the Future* (1975),[22] the Study Commission on Pharmacy called on pharmacy educators to develop competency-based curricula incorporating both the common and the differentiated knowledge and skills required for specific practice roles. The APhA-AACP-sponsored *National Study of the Practice of Pharmacy* (1979)[23] set forth standards of practice to assist curriculum committees in their efforts to design practice-oriented courses and help accrediting bodies evaluate educational programs. The APhA Task Force on Pharmacy Education (1984)[24] identified the competencies expected of the entry-level practitioner, endorsed the APhA-AACP practice standards, outlined curricular characteristics and a core curriculum, and recommended that the 6-year PharmD degree evolve "as the sole entry level for the practice of pharmacy."

In 1987 C. Douglas Hepler[21] articulated the concept of pharmaceutical care during a special session of the AACP annual meeting in Charleston, S.C., forcing pharmacy educators to view pharmaceutical education in a new light. Two years later, at the second Pharmacy in the 21st Century Conference, Hepler and Linda M. Strand[17] refined their pharmaceutical care concept into a new practice philosophy that captured the imagination of practitioners and educators alike. In July 1989 AACP president William A. Miller appointed a Commission to Implement Change in Pharmaceutical Education to articulate a mission of pharmacy practice that could serve as the basis for pharmaceutical education. "If we wish to develop the concept of pharmaceutical care, then we must produce pharmacists with sufficient knowledge and clinical experience to enable them to confidently assume responsibility for drug use control," Miller argued. "To achieve this goal will require more, not less, education and training."[25] Two months later, ACPE sent shock waves through the educational community by announcing its intention to evaluate and accredit the PharmD as "the only professional degree program" as early as 2000.[26] At the time, 42 of the nation's schools and colleges of pharmacy offered only the BS degrees, 22 offered both the BS and the PharmD degrees, and 10 offered only the PharmD degree.[27]

Over the next 3 years, the AACP Commission produced two background papers describing the mission of pharmaceutical education, its curricular content, educational outcomes, and processes and a position paper, "Entry-level Education in Pharmacy: A Commitment to Change,"[28] each of which was carefully scrutinized by the AACP Board of Directors and forwarded to its House of Delegates for action. On July 15, 1992, the House delegates approved 17 policy statements supporting "a single entry-level educational program at the doctoral level."[29]

After 42 years of debate, dissension, and division, American pharmaceutical education had finally passed a crucial decision point. Over the next decade, the nation's schools and colleges of pharmacy would face the challenge of implementing new educational programs to prepare America's pharmacists to provide pharmaceutical care into the next century.

This article originally appeared in *Journal of the American Pharmaceutical Association*, 42, no. 4 (July/Aug 2002): 542-44.

References

1. Richards RQ. Facing the second century: address of the president-elect. *J Am Pharm Assoc (Pract Pharm Ed)*. 1952;13:742.
2. Fischl LJ. Address of the chairman of the House of Delegates. *J Am Pharm Assoc (Pract Pharm Ed)*. 1952,13:736.
3. Blauch LE, Webster GL. *The Pharmaceutical Curriculum*. Washington, DC: American Council on Education; 1952.
4. Mrtek RG. Pharmaceutical education in these United States—an interpretive historical essay of the twentieth century. *Am J Pharm Educ* 1976;40.356(n 142), 357.
5. Holland MO. Enrollments in colleges. *Am Prof Pharm*. 1953;19(1):21.
6. Fischelis RP. Straight from headquarters: Eisenhower has the answer. *J Am Pharm Assoc* (Pract Pharm Ed). 1953;14:695.
7. Howe M. Report of Committee on Resolution. *Proc Natl Assoc Boards Pharm*. 1953; 49:176.

8. Convention recommendations and resolutions. *J Am Pharm Assoc* (Pract Pharm Ed). 1953;14:571.
9. Burt JB. Address of the president-elect. *Am J Pharm Educ.* 1954;18:573.
10. Deno RA. Summary of the executive session 1954 annual meeting, American Association of Colleges of Pharmacy. *Am J Pharm Educ.* 1954;18:674.
11. Buerki RA In search of excellence: the first century of the American Association of Colleges of Pharmacy. *Am J Pharm Educ.* 1999;63(fall suppl):74-81.
12. Rx sales outstrip US income growth *Drug Topics.* October 1949:1 -2.
13. Average doctor wrote 167 fewer Rxs in 1960 than in 1959, AD study shows. *American Druggist* March 1961:7.
14. Pharmaceutical Manufacturers Association. Prescription Drug Industry Fact Book. Washington, DC: Pharmaceutical Manufacturers Association; 1973:24, 31, 67.
15. Buerki RA, Vottero LD. *Ethical Responsibilities in Pharmacy Practice.* Rev. ed. Madison, Wisc: American Institute of the History of Pharmacy; 1996:19-21.
16. Kalman SH, Schlegel JF. Standards of practice for the profession of pharmacy. *Am Pharm* 1979:NS19:133-45.
17. Hepler CD, Strand LM. Opportunities and responsibilities in pharmaceutical care. *Am J Pharm Educ.* 1989;53(winter suppl):7S-1 5S.
18. Clark HT Jr. A challenge to American pharmacy. *J Am Pharm Assoc.* 1965:NS5:20.
19. Abrams RE. Education for a dynamic future. Paper presented at: Ohio State University: April 15, 1964: Columbus, Ohio. [Cited in: Parks LM. Pharmaceutical education for the future. *Am J Pharm Educ.* 1967:31 :23.]
20. Goyan JE. Pharmacy practice—structure and function. *Am J Pharm Educ.* 1974 38:693,
21. Hepler CD. The third wave in pharmaceutical education: the clinical movement. *Am J Pharm Educ.* 1987;51:369-85.
22. Study Commission on Pharmacy. *Pharmacists for the Future: The Report of the Study Commission on Pharmacy.* Ann Arbor, Mich: Health Administration Press; 1 975:141 -2.
23. Rosenfeld M, Thornton RF, Glazer R *A National Study of the Practice of Pharmacy.* Washington, DC: American Pharmaceutical Association; 1978.
24. Task Force on Pharmacy Education. *The professional practice degree. In: The Final Report of the Task Force on Pharmacy Education.* Washington, DC: American Pharmaceutical Association; 1984:25-8.
25. Miller WA Planning for pharmacy education in the 21st century: AACP's leadership role. *Am J Pharm Educ.* 1989;53:338.
26. Nona DA. Annual report of the American Council on Pharmaceutical Education to the profession and the public. *Am J Pharm Educ.* 1990 54:203.
27. Penna RP, Sherman MS. Enrollments in schools and colleges of pharmacy, 1989-1990. Table III. Full-time entry level programs (BS and PharmD). *Am J Pharm Educ.* 1990:54: 455-6.
28. Commission to Implement Change in Pharmaceutical Education. A position paper: entry-level education in pharmacy: A commitment to change. *Am J Pharm Educ.* 1993;57:366-74.
29. Sandmann RA. Chair report of the Bylaws and Policy Development Committee: policy statements. *Am J Pharm Educ.* 1992,66(winter suppl):13S-15S.

The Pharmaceutical Industry, 1852-1902

*by Dennis B. Worthen**

Fₒᵣ most of the first 200 years of European settlement on the northeast coast of America, little pharmaceutical manufacturing took place. Medications were either compounded from a limited number of drugs or imported from the continent as finished products, intermediates, or patent medicines. Manufacturing of medications was a cottage industry that served a limited number of customers in a small geographic area. The apothecary shops, frequently owned and operated by the physicians of the period, compounded medications for the use of that practitioner or for a few practitioners. The population was too scattered, and medical knowledge too sketchy and unstandardized, to warrant manufacturing on any appreciable scale.

At the beginning of the Revolutionary War, medical supplies came from individual apothecaries. However, since that system could not meet the demands of an army, Andrew Craigie's laboratory and storehouse were established in Carlisle, Pennsylvania, to supply medications to the military.[1,2] Thus the Revolutionary War provided an important stimulus to the manufacturing industry in North America, which grew slowly from this meager beginning.

Philadelphia was the cradle of American pharmacy.[3] Notable firsts for the city include the first hospital in 1751 (Pennsylvania Hospital), the first hospital pharmacy in 1752, and the first college of pharmacy (Philadelphia College of Pharmacy) in 1821. It also became one of the centers of pharmaceutical manufacturing. By 1786 Christopher Marshall, Jr., and Charles Marshall were manufacturing ammonium chloride and Glauber's Salt. In 1822 a firm that would later become Powers & Weightman began manufacturing quinine only 2 years after its isolation from cinchona bark. Other manufacturing concerns started in the corridor stretching from Philadelphia and Baltimore to New York and Boston. However, all of these manufacturing businesses remained small and regional.

---

*Dennis B. Worthen, PhD, is the Lloyd Scholar, Lloyd Library and Museum, Cincinnati, Ohio.

Rise of the Industry

Three factors gave rise to the American pharmaceutical manufacturing industry: the need for pure and standardized products, a distribution system for raw materials and finished goods, and a sizable population. By the time the American Pharmaceutical Association (APhA) was established in 1852, each of these factors was in place.

The lack of pure and unadulterated products was a concern. In response to imported crude drugs that were "substituted, adulterated or deficient in strength,"[4] pharmacists and physicians petitioned Congress to enact a law prohibiting the importation of medications of inferior quality. Such a law was passed, and its enforcement begun in 1848. However, it was largely ineffective, since the inspectors were political appointees rather than trained observers and were unable to identify adulterated products. It was problems with adulteration and quality that led to the formation of APhA.

The United States was growing both in population and physical mass. In 1825 the Erie Canal began operating from Albany to Buffalo, opening the heartland of the country to immigrants arriving in New York. The first railroads were under construction in the 1820s and 1830s, and by the beginning of the Civil War there were more than 30,000 miles of rail in the country. In 1869, at Promontory, Utah, the transcontinental railroad joined East and

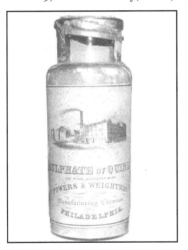

West. The population soared from a little less than 4 million in 1790 at the first census to more than 23 million in 1850.[5] A market of significant size was available, and the means to move raw materials to manufacturers and finished products to consumers were in place. In 1850 California was admitted to the union as the 31st state. The time was ripe for pharmaceutical manufacturing to move from a cottage industry to an organized industry. The emerging industry was inexorably linked with the emerging profession; both were born as a consequence of the need for quality and the expectations of an expanding market.

Even as APhA was being established in 1852, Powers & Weightman of Philadelphia was already producing Sulphate of Quinine as shown here.

Patent Medicines

The 19th century saw the emergence of the American patent medicine industry. (The term patent medicine is not used in the modern sense, because a patent did not cover these products—although manufacturers made exorbitant health claims for them, and their ingredients were kept secret.) Several factors supported the rapid growth of this industry. First was a growing distrust of the physicians of the day and their cures. Physicians were few and far between, and their fees were frequently much higher than patients wished to pay. Moreover, the cures physicians offered—bloodletting, violent purging, and use of calomel—often were worse than the disease. Patent medicines, on the other hand, were easy to come by. They were available in every type of mercantile establishment, and they were sold almost at the patient's door by all kinds of traveling shows. Not only did consumers get their medications, they were also entertained in the bargain. However, many of these products were little more than alcohol, water, and flavoring, in spite of the outrageous claims of therapeutic benefit.

The growth of the patent medicine industry was greatly enhanced by advertising. Newspaper ads, almanacs, and traveling shows were just a few of the methods used to reach the unwary public. Many manufacturers used personal testimonials as proof of effectiveness: others, such as Lydia Pinkham, used personal responses to letters from sufferers as a way to disseminate the product message.

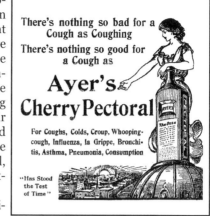

There's nothing so bad for a Cough as Coughing

There's nothing so good for a Cough as

Ayer's Cherry Pectoral

For Coughs, Colds, Croup, Whooping-cough, Influenza, la Grippe, Bronchitis, Asthma, Pneumonia, Consumption

"Has Stood the Test of Time"

Apothecary James Cook Ayer of Lowell, Massachusetts, first marketed Ayer's Cherry Pectoral in 1841. Ayer refused to disclose the formula, and it was later found to include morphine, tartar emetic, and ipecac, dissolved in syrup of wild cherry.

One of the first acts of the newly formed APhA was to condemn the use of these nostrums. Over the next half century, the battle with nostrum peddlers was a continuing saga that finally culminated in the passage of the Pure Food and Drug Act of 1906.

Emergence of an Eponymous Industry

The Civil War marked the emergence of the manufacturing industry. Again, the impetus was the needs of armies of vast numbers of men. Several companies, such as Frederick Stearns and E. R. Squibb & Sons, were established before the war and were major providers of medications to the Union forces. Veterans, such as Eli Lilly, a former colonel in the Indiana artillery, formed other companies after the war.

Pharmacists, including John Wyeth, William Warner, and Louis Dohme, and physicians, including Walter Abbott and William E. Upjohn, founded most manufacturing companies of the period. The company bore the name of the founder; this eponymous nature was particularly important for the medications of the day. Ostensibly, the name and reputation of individuals were sufficient testimony that the products contained the ingredients as labeled. Indeed, many companies provided the same product, produced in the same manner; only the name of Lilly, Squibb, or Wyeth differentiated one manufacturer's goods from another's.

There was innovation in the period, usually in the dosage form offered. William Warner began his company to produce the first sugar-coated pills, while Upjohn began producing the first compressed friable pills. Lilly started with a line of fluid extracts and syrups. John Uri Lloyd and his brothers be-

Pharmaceutical Company Founding Dates	
Frederick Stearns & Company	1855
William R. Warner & Co.	1856
E. R. Squibb & Sons	1858
Reed & Carnrick	1860
Wyeth	1860
Sharp & Dohme	1860
Burroughs Bros Manufacturing Company	1863
Parke, Davis & Company	1866
Lloyd Brothers	1870
Chilcott Laboratories	1875
Eli Lilly & Company	1876
Lambert Company	1884
Norwich Eaton	1885
Johnson & Johnson	1885
Upjohn Company	1886
Armour Pharmaceuticals	1886
Bristol-Myers	1887
Merck (U.S.)	1887
Abbott Laboratories	1888
G. D. Searle	1888
Becton Dickinson	1897

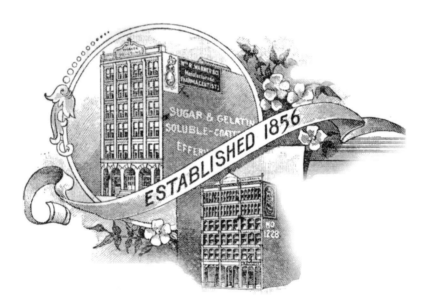

Philadelphia community pharmacist William R. Warner pioneered the mass production of sugar-coated pills designed to "mask the taste of disagreeable medicines."

gan producing "specifics" for the eclectic physicians of the period.

Combination

The manufacturing industry and APhA were closely linked during the last half of the 19th century. Many of the founders of the early houses were pharmacists and served as APhA officers. There was a mutual interest in providing suitable medicinal products that were unadulterated. Indeed, it was a time when two branches of pharmacy, practice and manufacturing, were joined in the provision of medications to an expanding nation.

This article originally appeared in *Journal of the American Pharmaceutical Association,* 40, no.5 (Sept/Oct 2000): 589-91.

References

1. Griffenhagen GB. *Drug Supplies in the American Revolution.* United States National Museum Bulletin 225. Washington, DC: Smithsonian Institution; 1961.
2. Cowen DL. *The Colonial and Revolutionary Heritage of Pharmacy in America.* Trenton, New Jersey Pharmaceutical Association;1976.
3. Mahoney T. *Merchants of Life.* New York, NY: Harper Brothers;1959:30.
4. Sonnedecker G. *Kremers and Urdang's History of Pharmacy.* Fourth edition. Philadelphia, Pa: J.B. Lippincott Co;1976:198.
5. *Study 00003: Historical Demographic Economic, and Social Data: U.S., 1790-1970.* Ann Arbor, Mich: Inter-University Consortium for Political and Social Research; 1979.

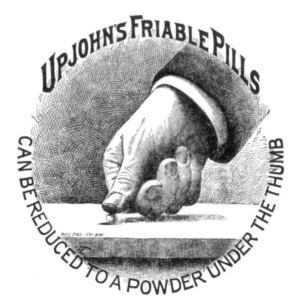

The Upjohn Pill and Granule Co. of Kalamazoo, Michigan, patented Upjohn's Friable Pills in 1885 as "capable of being crushed and powdered under the thumb." In 1902 the firm became known as the Upjohn Company.

The Pharmaceutical Industry, 1902-1952

by Dennis B. Worthen*

At the beginning of the 20th century, the pharmaceutical manufacturing industry consisted mostly of small and regional companies; only a few manufacturers, such as Eli Lilly and Squibb, had a national presence. It was manufacturing prowess rather than research that characterized the industry. Mahoney offered some facts that place the lack of concentration and size in the American industry in perspective: 3,512 firms failed between 1932 and 1934 at the height of the Great Depression; in 1939 no single ethical drug manufacturer had a sales volume as great as Macy's in New York or Hudson's in Detroit; and the total sales volume for all 1,100 pharmaceutical companies was $150 million at the manufacturing level.[1]

Era of Biologicals

The end of the 19th century and the beginning of the 20th century saw the rise of biologicals as an important part of the pharmaceutical industry. The discovery of some causative agents of disease and the emerging science of bacteriology ushered in the era of biologicals. In the last decade of the 19th century diphtheria and tetanus antitoxins were prepared in laboratories in France and Germany. Perhaps the most important product of the period was antidiphtheria serum; it was an effective therapy for one of the most feared childhood diseases of the day. In 1894 the H.K. Mulford Company established the first biologicals laboratory in America in Philadelphia for the production of a reliable antitoxin.[2] By 1895 the New York City Board of Health Laboratories was producing diphtheria antitoxin, as were health departments in other cities, including those in St. Louis, Cincinnati, and Boston.

In 1901 tragedy struck in St. Louis when at least five children died of tetanus after they received contaminated diphtheria antitoxin that had been produced by the city's health department. Apparently, this situation was not unique. In Camden, N.J., numerous cases of tetanus were reported in chil-

---

*Dennis B. Worthen, PhD, is the Lloyd Scholar, Lloyd Library and Museum, Cincinnati, Ohio.

dren who had been vaccinated for smallpox, and isolated reports were received from other American and European cities.

Ultimately, the need to regulate the interstate sale of viruses, serums, toxins, and analogous products led the U.S. Congress to pass the Biologics Control Act of 1902. President Theodore Roosevelt signed this first federal pharmaceutical law 4 years before the passage of the Pure Food and Drug Act, placing the production of biological products under the control of the forerunner of today's Public Health Service.[3]

Parke, Davis & Company and H.K. Mulford were among the first companies to produce biologics commercially. In 1902 Parke Davis would receive the first license to manufacture biologics and Mulford the second. Ernst Joseph Lederle resigned his position as director of the New York Health Department to establish Lederle Antitoxin Laboratories in 1906, and received biologics license Number 17.[4]

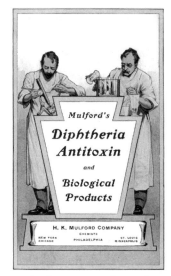

Mulford was an early producer of diphtheria antitoxin in the United States. Mulford would become part of Sharp & Dohme in 1929. Photo courtesy of the AIHP Kremers Reference Files.

Food and Drugs Act

The food and drug law of 1906 was passed primarily to control problems in the food production industry. The law was expanded to cover drugs when the government could no longer ignore problems in the proprietary pharmaceutical industry. However, the law's requirements only applied to interstate violations when a product was misbranded or adulterated. Harvey W. Wiley's Bureau of Chemistry in the U.S. Department of Agriculture was given responsibility for enforcing the act. The Shirley Amendment of 1912 added the requirement that labels could not contain any therapeutic statement "which is false and fraudulent."[5] The large, reputable national companies with analytical laboratories were largely unaffected by the regulations and were, in fact, generally in favor of the regulations that were intended to curb abuses that discredited the industry.[6]

Table 1. Companies Attending the First Meeting of the American Association of Pharmaceutical Chemists, Detroit, 1910

Abbott Alkaloid Co. (Chicago, IL)	G. D. Searle & Co. (Chicago, IL)
Columbus Pharmacal Co. (Columbus, OH)	Stearns & White Co. (Chicago, IL)
J. F. Hartz Co. (Detroit, MI)	R. J. Strasenburgh Co. (Rochester, NY)
Howard-Hold Co. (Cedar Rapids, IA)	Toledo Pharmacal Co. (Toledo, OH)
Maltbie Chemical Co. (Newark, NJ)	Truax, Green & Co. (Chiacago, IL)
Norwich Pharmacal Co. (Norwich, NY)	Webster, Warnock Co. (Memphis, TN)
O. F. Schmid Chemical Co. (Jackson, MI)	Zemmer Co. (Pittsburgh, PA)
Pitman, Myers & Co (Indianapolis, IN)	

source:-reference 7

Associations of Pharmaceutical Manufacturers

Partly in response to increasing regulation and the need to share information, manufacturers began to establish separate organizations, although many individuals maintained their membership and leadership in the American Pharmaceutical Association. In 1910 the first American association of pharmaceutical manufacturers, the American Association of Pharmaceutical Chemists, was formed in Detroit. The original members were mostly small, family-owned companies (see Table 1).[7] At the Association's fourth meeting in 1913, a nascent code of ethics was shared, and Charles Wesley Dunn, a New York attorney and expert on the Food and Drugs Act, was retained to advise the association on the new regulations. The name of the organization was changed to American Pharmaceutical Manufacturers Association in 1922. In 1912 a second organization was formed in New York. The National Association of Manufacturers of Medicinal Products (NAMMP) (see Table 2) had a distinctly different type of membership, although there was some overlap.[8] In 1916 the NAMMP changed its name to American Drug Manufacturers Association. Both organizations provided a forum for the exchange of information on common problems, such as tariffs, legislation and regulation, and the promotion of high standards in manufacturing.

Federal Food, Drug and Cosmetic Act of 1938

The Food and Drug Administration was formed out of the predecessor Bureau of Chemistry in 1931. In the following years there were attempts to pass new legislation that would plug the loopholes and strengthen the penalties of the 1906 act. However, these efforts received little congressional support until another tragedy struck. Intending to introduce a liquid form of sulfanilamide, Massengill, an old and respected firm, determined that diethylene glycol was a satisfactory solvent. The company began selling Elixir of Sulfanilamide without testing it; a number of people, mostly children, died as a consequence of the solvent's toxicity. Under the 1906 law Massengill could only be prosecuted for mislabeling the product as an elixir, since it contained no alcohol. The public outcry provided the impetus for the passage of the Food, Drug and Cosmetic Act of 1938.

The new law required that manufacturers prove a product was safe before it could be placed into interstate commerce. Importantly, it also established the requirement for adequate labeling, which in turn led to the distinction between products that could be used only on a physician's prescription and those that could be adequately labeled for self-medication.[9]

Research and Development

The American pharmaceutical industry of the early 20th century was predominantly a manufacturing industry. Individual companies started by serving a geographical region with an assorted line of standard products or by championing a specific dosage form or manufacturing process. The catalogs of the larger manufacturers ran to several hundred pages, and some pharmacies would identify themselves as a supplier of Squibb products or those of Lilly, Wyeth, or Parke-Davis. When one company brought a new product to market, it could be quickly copied and supplied by a number of other companies. Innovation was not characteristic of the industry.

World War I brought considerable changes to the pharmaceutical industry in the United States. A number of German products had been patented and were being produced in the United States under licensing arrangements. American scientists broke German patents for essential products, such as salvarsan, procaine, and barbital. At the conclusion of the war, some foreign assets were seized by the Alien Property Custodian and auctioned. Sterling acquired the rights to the Bayer aspirin trademark through this process.

A number of companies started doing research, first to differentiate themselves from other producers and later to develop new products. At the beginning, research was largely limited to substantiating claims of quality, purity, and assay. Lilly, Merck, Squibb, and others would later establish their own research institutes, which functioned as hybrid organizations pursuing both pure and applied research. However, with few exceptions, such as insulin, the major sources of research were European companies and institutions and American academic institutions. This situation changed after World War II.[10]

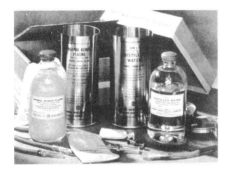

Plasma administration units consisted of two vacuum-sealed cans, one containing plasma and the second a bottle of sterile distilled water, in a waterproofed box along with all of the necessary tubing and needles for administration. Photo courtesy of the Lloyd Library, Cincinnati, Ohio. Source: Reference 13

World War II

At the beginning of World War II the United States was again dependent on other countries for essential raw materials and medicines. The world supply of medicinal grade quinine passed to the control of the Japanese in 1941. I.G. Farben patented Atabrine (quinacrine), a synthetic alternative to quinine, in 1932 and supplied the chemical intermediates to Winthrop for final production with the threat of war in 1940. Winthrop scientists learned how to make the product from raw material available in the United States and subsequently provided millions of Atabrine tablets for Allied forces fighting in malaria-ridden areas.[11]

Pharmaceutical manufacturers worked together and with the government on a number of projects in support of the war effort. The two most notable examples were the production of dried plasma and penicillin. Building on basic research by academics and clinicians on blood and its constituents, the industry was able to devise techniques and equipment to produce millions of units of dried plasma from blood collected by the American Red Cross. By the end of the war the American Red Cross had collected more than 13 million pints of blood, most of which was processed into dried plasma and packaged for military use. Thirteen pharmaceutical companies (Abbott, Armour, Ben Venue, Cutter, Hyland, Lederle, Lilly, Parke-Davis, Reichel, Sharp & Dohme, Squibb, Upjohn, and Wyeth) were involved in processing dried plasma and albumin for the military during the war; Lilly alone processed more than two million units of dried plasma.

Penicillin was another triumph of teamwork. Initially research was undertaken by a group of three East Coast companies (Merck, Pfizer, and Squibb), but a group of companies based in the Midwest (Abbott, Lilly, Parke-Davis, and Upjohn) quickly added their efforts, as did three companies unaffiliated with either group (Lederle, Reichel Laboratories, and Heyden Chemical). In 1943 total production was 425 million units, and distribution was limited to the military. In 1944 the War Production Board signed contracts with six companies (Ben Venue, Cheplin, Commercial Solvents, Cutter, Sterling, and Wyeth) to boost production, and in May the Board established a civilian distribution mechanism. In June 1945 alone, 646 billion units were produced.[12]

Postwar Industry

For the American pharmaceutical industry, the postwar period was one of expansion, fueled largely by the rapid discovery and launch of new compounds. Streptomycin (Merck, 1945), chlortetracycline (Lederle, 1948), and chloramphenicol (Parke-Davis, 1949) were the first results of a vigorous search for broad-spectrum antibiotics. Benadryl (Parke-Davis, 1946) was the first marketed antihistamine. Tubocurarine chloride, a muscle relaxant (Squibb, 1946), and thrombin, a hemostatic resulting from the blood research during the war (Upjohn, 1946), were new surgical adjuncts. This was the beginning of the period when miracles were expected and extolled to health professionals and consumers alike.

APhA Leadership

Throughout the first 50 years of the 20th century, relationships between the pharmaceutical manufacturing industry and APhA remained strong. Two presidents of the association were from the industry, Alfred Dohme (1917-1918) and H.A.B. Dunning (1929-1930) (see Figure 4). Four honorary APhA presidents-Edward Mallinckrodt (1927-1928), Henry Wellcome (1931-1932), Josiah Lilly Sr. (1934-1935), and Gustavus Pfeiffer (1947-1948)-came from industry, as did four Remington medallists-John Uri Lloyd (1920), H.A.B. Dunning (1926), Henry Wellcome (1934) and Josiah Lilly Sr. (1942).

This article originally appeared in *Journal of the American Pharmaceutical Association,* 41, no. 5 (Sept/Oct 2001):656-59.

References

1.   Mahoney T. *Merchants of Life.* New York, NY: Harper & Brothers; 1959:4.
2.   H.K. Mulford Company. *Diphtheria Antitoxic Serum.* 7th edition. Philadelphia, Pa: H.K. Mulford Company; 1897.
3.   Kondratas R. Biologics Control Act of 1902. In: Young JH, ed. *The Early Years of Federal*

Food and Drug Control. Madison, Wisc: American Institute of the History of Pharmacy; 1982:7-27.

4. Mahoney T. *Merchants of Life*. New York, NY: Harper & Brothers; 1959:163.

5. Temin P. *Taking Your Medicine: Drug Regulation in the United States*. Cambridge, Mass: Harvard University Press; 1980:33.

6. Liebenau, J. *Medical Science and Medical Industry: The Formation of the American Pharmaceutical Industry*. Baltimore, Md: Johns Hopkins University Press; 1987:94-95.

7. Maltbie, B.L. *A Quarter Century of Progress in Manufacturing Pharmacy*. New York, NY: American Pharmaceutical Manufacturers Association; 1937.

8. National Association of Manufacturers of Medicinal Products. *Proceedings of the First Annual Meeting of National Association of Manufacturers of Medicinal Products*. New York, NY: NAMMP; 1913.

9. Temin P. *Taking Your Medicine: Drug Regulation in the United States*. Cambridge, Mass: Harvard University Press; 1980:47.

10. Swann JP. *Academic Scientists and the Pharmaceutical Industry*. Baltimore, MD: Johns Hopkins Press; 1988.

11. Sonnedecker G. *Kremers and Urdangs History of Pharmacy*. 3rd ed. Philadelphia. Pa.: J.B. Lippincott; 1963:292.

12. Helfand WH, Woodruff HB, Coleman KMH, Cowen DL. Wartime industrial penicillin in the United States. In: Parascandola J, ed. *The History of Antibiotics: A Symposium*. Madison, Wisc: American Institute for the History of Pharmacy; 1980: 31-56.

13. *Therapeutic Notes*. January 1943: 13.

Table 2. Original Roll of Membership of the National Association of Manufacturers of Medicinal Products, New York, 1912

Abbott Alkaloid Co. (Chicago, IL)
Allaire, Woodward & Co. (Peoria, PA)
Armour & Co. (Chicago, IL)
Bauer & Black (Chicago, IL)
Farbenfabriken (Elberfeld, Germany)[a]
Hance Bros. & White (Philadelphia, PA)
Heyden Chemical Works (New York, NY)
Johnson & Johnson[b] (New Brunswick, NJ)
Lilly & Co. (Eli) (Indianapolis, IN)
Mallinckrodt Chemical Works (St. Louis, MO)
Merck & Co. (New York, NY)
Merrill [sic] Chemical Co., (William S.) (Cincinnati, OH)
Monsanto Chemical Works (St. Louis, MO)
Mulford Co. (H. K.) (Philadelphia, PA)
Nelson, Baker & Co. (Detroit, MI)
Norwich Pharmacal Co. (Norwich, NY)
Parke, Davis & Co. (Detroit, MI)
Patch Co. (E. L.) (Boston, MA)
Pfizer & Co. (Charles) (New York, NY)
Pitman-Myers (Indianapolis, IN)
Powers-Weightman-Rosengarten Co. (Philadelphia, PA)
Roessler & Hasslacher Chemical Co.[b] (New York, NY)
Schaefer Alkaloid Works (Maywood, NJ)
Seabury & Johnson (New York, NY)
Sharp & Dohme (Baltimore, MD)
Sorby Vaccine Co.[a] (Chicago, IL)
Stearns & Co. (Frederick) (Detroit, MI)
Thayer & Co. (Henry) (Cambridge, Boston, MA)
Tilden Co. (New Lebanon, NY)
Upjohn Co. (Kalamazoo, MI)
Wampole Co. (Henry K.) (Philadelphia, PA)
Warner & Co. (William R.) (Philadelphia, PA)

[a]Listed in the roll in the proceedings of the association's first annual meeting but not in the alphabethical list of companies
[b]Listed in the alphabetical list of companies but not in the roll.

The Pharmaceutical Industry, 1952-2002

by Dennis B. Worthen*

T HE history of the pharmaceutical industry in the United States during the last half of the 20th century was characterized by a number of broad and interrelated trends, including research, organizational and market shifts, and consolidation and expansion.

Composition of the Industry

At the beginning of the postwar period, the industry was made up of a large number of relatively small pharmaceutical "houses," as they were then called. Many of these firms still had members of the founding families involved in the business. Some companies, such as Cutter laboratories and G.D. Searle, were "specialty" houses that focused their marketing and research efforts by therapeutic category or geographic region. Other firms, such as Eli Lilly, Parke-Davis, and E.R. Squibb, were "full-line houses" that marketed a broad array of products, often internationally. In addition to the traditional pharmaceutical manufacturers, firms that had focused on proprietary preparations or chemicals in the earlier part of the century moved into clinical research and production of prescription products. Bristol Laboratories, largely known for such proprietaries as the laxative Sal-Hepatica and Ipana toothpaste, entered the ethical[a] field with the purchase of Cheplin Laboratories. Norwich Pharmacal started its own research arm, Eaton laboratories, and Pfizer moved from manufacturing chemicals to manufacturing pharmaceuticals.

---

*Dennis B. Worthen, PhD, is the Lloyd Scholar, Lloyd Library and Museum, Cincinnati, Ohio.
[a] "Ethical" products were those that were promoted only to physicians and, to a lesser extent, pharmacists.

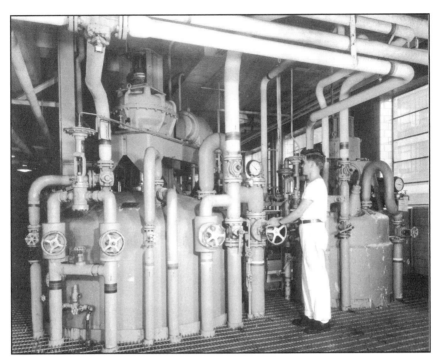

Pharmaceutical manufacturing came of age during the period 1952-2002, when the latest drugs were developed and produced in enormous quantities.

Research

During World War II, the Committee on Medical Research of the Office of Scientific Research and Development (OSRD) sponsored research in a number of areas that had military importance, including blood products, antiinfectives, antimalarials, and steroids. For example, in reaction to a 1941 report of enhanced endurance by German fighter pilots, OSRD led an innovative and cooperative research program on corticosteroids that included Merck, the Mayo Clinic, and several universities.[1] Innovative research during the war was marked by such cooperation among companies, academia, and the government. As a consequence of this environment of opportunity, many companies invested heavily in research and built the necessary infrastructures, including sales and marketing, to take advantage of new discoveries in life sciences and technologies in the postwar world.[2]

Achilladelis divided the progress of industry-supported research into three distinct phases.[3] The first phase (1930-1960) encompassed the watershed years of the war technologies. This phase was characterized by increasing in-house research; the major therapeutic categories were vitamins, sulfas, antibiotics, antihistamines, and hormones. The second phase (1960-1980) was a period of industry maturation. Research attention shifted from treating diseases caused by organisms to correcting problems associated with heredity, diet, and environment. Breakthrough products included the first oral contraceptives, nonsteroidal anti-inflammatories, the cephalosporins, and the anxiolytics beginning with Librium. The current phase (beginning in 1980) is characterized by globalization, biotechnology, and the phenomenon of blockbusters—those products with sales exceeding a half billion dollars a year. The first to reach this plateau was Smith Kline & French's Tagamet.[3] During this period, pharmaceutical companies have shifted their research focus from organic chemistry to the life sciences, especially molecular biology.[4]

The pharmaceutical industry is deeply rooted in the sciences. The National Science Foundation reported in 1967 that 156 of every 1,000 employees in the pharmaceutical industry were scientists. The chemical industry had the next highest numbers, with 48 out of 1,000 employees being scientists. Scientists numbered 32 out of 1,000 employees in the petroleum industry, and the average for all manufacturing industries was 8 out of 1,000.[5] These proportions were holding steady as late as 1998, when the pharmaceutical industry accounted for over 18% of all company-funded basic research and 4.8% of all research scientists and engineers.[6] In the years between 1980 and 2000 pharmaceutical research and development expenditures increased from almost $2 billion to over $26 billion. To place these numbers in context, in 2000 the total budget of the National Institutes of Health was less than $18 billion.[7]

In the first half of the 20th century, the major manufacturers belonged to either the American Pharmaceutical Manufacturers Association or the American Drug Manufacturers Association. By the early 1950s many companies belonged to both organizations, and the overlap in focus had become an issue. In 1958 the two organizations merged into the Pharmaceutical Manufacturers Association (PMA). In 1994 PMA changed its name to Pharmaceutical Research and Manufacturers of America (PhRMA).

Multisource Products

Until the emergence of the research-intensive pharmaceutical industry in the post-World War II period, most medicinal products were multisourced. Manufacturers were free to produce, under their own brand names, any line of products appearing in the *United States Pharmacopoeia* or the *National Formulary*. Pharmacists had a great deal of latitude to decide whether they would be distributors for Parke-Davis, Squibb, or Lilly.

By the early 1950s, in response to counterfeiting problems, states passed antisubstitution laws that required pharmacists to dispense exactly what physicians had written. Pharmacists could select products only when physicians wrote prescription orders using generic names. In 1953 the National Pharmaceutical Council was formed by 12 research-intensive manufacturers to support the antisubstitution effort.

Repeal of the state antisubstitution laws was largely fueled by economic concerns. On one level, the government, as a purchaser of medications, sought lower prices for its programs. On a second level, community pharmacists were also seeking ways to lower the costs of stocking multiple brands of the same products. In 1974 Michigan became the first state to repeal its antisubstitution law; by 1980, 45 states permitted substitution. In spite of the repeals, substitution was not popular with physicians, patients, or pharmacists.[8]

The generic pharmaceutical industry is made up of companies that are either subsidiaries of research-intensive companies or independent companies that manufacture or market only generic drugs. Growth in both the number of companies and sales volume can be attributed in large part to the 1984 passage of the Drug Price Competition and Patent Term Restoration Act, also known as the Waxman-Hatch Act. The law's modification and simplification of the Abbreviated New Drug Application (ANDA) process made it easier for generic manufacturers to enter the pharmaceutical market. The act also extended part of the patent exclusivity period that innovative manufacturers lost due to delays in U.S. Food and Drug Administration (FDA) approval of their products.[8-13]

Three trade associations represented the generic drug industry until 2000. That year, the Generic Pharmaceutical Industry Association and the National Pharmaceutical Alliance merged to form a new umbrella association, the Generic Pharmaceutical Association (GPhA). The National Association of Pharmaceutical Manufacturers joined GPhA in 2001.

Regulation

This 50-year period opened with the passage of the Humphrey-Durham Amendment to the Food, Drug and Cosmetic Act (FD&C Act) in 1952. Whereas the original FD&C Act established the basic requirement for proof of safety, Humphrey-Durham took the concept one step further. Products that were determined to need professional judgment for safe use were to be available by prescription; products that could be labeled so that they could be safely used by the public were to be available without a prescription. The amendment had considerable ramifications for pharmacy practice, particularly with regard to pharmacists' ability to refill prescriptions. It also had a significant impact on the pharmaceutical industry, as it established two categories of medications in the United States—prescription and nonprescription—and began the codification of the basis for distinguishing between the two classes.

The Drug Amendments of 1962 have been characterized as the "greatest force in the federal regulation of pharmaceutical products since the enactment of the 1906 Food and Drugs Act."[14] As a consequence of the thalidomide tragedy, the congressional scrutiny that began in 1959 with the Kefauver hearings on pricing and marketing practices culminated in a series of sweeping regulatory changes with the 1962 passage of the Kefauver-Harris Drug Amendments. Major changes included requiring manufacturers to provide substantial evidence of effectiveness in order to receive FDA approval for marketing a new medication and delegating oversight of new product testing to FDA; the manufacturer had to have FDA's approval to undertake the testing required for a New Drug Application. The 1962 amendments also established the requirements for good manufacturing practices and authorized FDA to do plant inspections. FDA was also authorized to remove products already on the market if they were unsafe or if there was a lack of scientific evidence for their effectiveness. FDA contracted with the National Research Council (NRC) to review all of the products that were marketed after the adoption of the 1938 safety requirements. Drugs marketed before 1938 were grandfathered, or exempted from the study. The NRC study, titled the Drug

Efficacy Study Implementation (DESI), led to the removal of a large number of ineffective products from the market. When the evidence was insufficient to make a determination of a product's safety or efficacy, FDA provided the manufacturer with the opportunity to develop new evidence.[15]

After the passage of the Waxman-Hatch Act in 1984, the generic industry grew quickly. The greatest economic success went to the company that was the first to receive an approved ANDA for its generic product. This race to be first led to the generic drug scandal in 1989, when generic manufacturers were caught bribing personnel in FDA's Office of Generic Drugs and falsifying data in ANDA submissions. FDA launched an internal investigation, and, eventually, individuals from the agency and several companies were tried and found guilty of fraud. Congress reacted with the passage of the Generic Drug Enforcement Act in 1992, which allowed FDA to debar companies guilty of fraud.[8-13]

The New Industry—Biotechnology

The American biotechnology industry formed independently of the established pharmaceutical industry. Frequently, companies were started by individual university-based scientists working in the area of molecular biology and funded by grants for basic research. The first biotech companies with a pharmaceutical focus were Genentech (established in 1976), Biogen (1978), Amgen (1980), and Immunex (1981). Several of the early companies followed the strategy of discovering, developing, producing, and marketing their own products; other companies focused on product discovery and development and licensing one of the existing pharmaceutical companies to produce and market the new medications. Some biotech companies that started out by licensing their products matured over time into pharmaceutical companies in their own right by adding sales and marketing infrastructures to the research base. Genentech, for example, focused its early research on growth hormones and insulin. In 1982, working with Lilly, Amgen received marketing approval for its first human medicine, Humulin (human insulin). By 1997 there were almost 400 biotechnology companies involved in the discovery and development of human medications, with over 500 compounds in the works. Approximately 10% of the sales of therapeutic agents in the United States were for biotechnology-derived products.[16]

Mergers and Acquisitions

Mergers and acquisitions have been part of the pharmaceutical industry from the beginning of its existence in the United States. The practice continued as the industry shifted from producing commodity products to developing and marketing innovative, unique products. For example, in 1946 William Warner and Company announced its intention to discontinue production of all "standard pharmaceuticals and galenicals" and concentrate on ethical products.[17] In 1952 this strategy was fully accomplished with the purchase of Chilcott Labs, a manufacturer of ethical pharmaceuticals. Companies also increased their business by cross-licensing innovative products discovered in other countries for distribution in the United States. For example, the French company Rhone Poulenc licensed its early phenothiazines,

Thorazine and Compazine, to Smith Kline & French and its antihistamine, Phenergan, to American Home Products.[18]

The merger activity was largely horizontal, as companies sought alliances that would expand skill sets such as research or marketing, allow them to grow from a regional to a national or international presence, or provide for a broader product line. Not all merger activity was restricted to health care business, however. Some corporations used a diversification strategy that would help stabilize business demands over a period of time. For example, Abbott purchased Faultless Rubber in 1966. Faultless made a broad array of products, including surgical gloves and catheters, as well as golf balls and golf clubs. In 1968 Squibb was spun off from its then parent Olin Matheson and merged with Beechnut, manufacturer of gum and Life Savers. In 1969 Upjohn acquired Homemakers Inc to provide home health care.

In the 1990s the traditional roles of the physician and pharmacist as the decision makers in the process of product selection were once again shifting with the growing influence of managed care and pharmacy benefits managers. One approach to managing this shift was the vertical integration of manufacturers with prescription plan companies. In 1993 Merck acquired Medco, and in 1994 SmithKlineBeecham acquired Diversified Pharmaceutical Services and Lilly acquired Pharmaceutical Card System. These acquisitions were viewed negatively by many, and by 1999 both Lilly and SmithKlineBeecham had divested.

The emergence of the new corporate entities often signaled a move away from eponymous firms that were closely connected by experience and history with the practice of pharmacy and medicine. No longer are many of the companies identified with the founder's name or place of founding; new names with little connection to their beginnings have emerged, such as Aventis and Novartis, or elided past the point of quick recognition, such as GlaxoSmithKline and AstraZeneca. Names of older companies, such as Hynson Westcott & Dunning, Sharp & Dohme, Vick Chemical, and A.H. Robins, have slowly disappeared or, if still in use, are linked to a specialty division or a product line.

Industry and the Pharmacy Profession

One of the continuing consequences of the controversy over generic drugs in the latter half of the 20th century has been the schism between the pharmaceutical industry and practitioners. The issues that surfaced around product selection clearly demonstrated that the two groups had different vested interests when it came to that question, in spite of a common heritage and many common concerns and values. The makeup of industry executives changed; few pharmacists rose to the chief executive level as the century progressed. No chief executive officers of industry were elected APhA president, as had been the case in the past, but two professional relations managers served as APhA president. These were 1956-1957 APhA president John A. MacCartney, who was professional relations manager of Parke, Davis and Company, and 1961-1962 APhA president, J. Warren Landsowne, who was professional relations manager of Eli Lilly & Company. Four chief executive officers of industry were elected honorary president: Eli Lilly (1953-1954), Fred Nitardy (1956-1957), E. Claiborne Robins (1992-1993), and Ernest Mario

(2002). A number of pharmacists who had served as APhA president later became industry executives: Jacob Miller (1978-1979), Herb Carlin (1984), and Marily Rhudy (1991-1992). Four Remington Medalists hailed from industry during the period: Eli Lilly (1958), Robert Hardt (1964), Ko Kuei Chen (1965), and Joseph Williams (1980). Jere Goyan, the 1992 Remington medalist, served as the only pharmacist head of FDA and later joined the biotechnology industry as an executive. Lawrence Weaver (1989) and Maurice Bectel (1996) joined PMA and its foundation as executives after their careers as educator and practitioner, respectively.

This article originally appeared in *Journal of the American Pharmaceutical Association,* 42, no. 5 (Sept/Oct 2002): 683-86.

References

1. Mahoney T. *The Merchants of Life.* New York, NY: Harper;1959:198.
2. Landau R, Achilladelis B, Scriabine A, eds. *Pharmaceutical Innovation: Revolutionizing Human Health.* Philadelphia, Pa: Chemical Heritage Foundation; 1999:79.
3. Achilladelis B. Innovation in the pharmaceutical industry. In: Landau R, Achilladelis B Scriabine A, eds. *Pharmaceutical Innovation: Revolutionizing Human Health.* Philadelphia, Pa: Chemical Heritage Foundation; 1999:123.
4. Achilladelis B. Innovation in the pharmaceutical industry. In: Landau R, Achilladelis B; Scriabine A, eds. *Pharmaceutical Innovation: Revolutionizing Human Health.* Philadelphia, Pa: Chemical Heritage Foundation, 1999:1147.
5. Scheele LM. The role of industry in an accelerated national program of biomedical drug development. In: *Research in the Service of Man: Biomedical Knowledge Development, and Use.* Report prepared for: Committee on Government Operations, U.S. Senate, 90th Cong, 1st sess: 1967.
6. *The Critical Roles of R&D in the Development of New Drugs.* Washington, DC: PriceWaterhouseCoopers 2001. Cited by: *Pharmaceutical/ Industry Profile 2002.* Washington, DC: Pharmaceutical Research and Manufacturers of America; 2002.
7. *Pharmaceutical Industry Profile 2002.* Washington, DC: Pharmaceutical Research and Manufacturers of America; 2002:12.
8. Ascione FJ, Kirking DM, Gaither CA, Welage LS. Historical overview of generic medication policy. *J Am Pharm Assoc.* 2001 ;41: 567-77.
9. Kirking DM. Perspectives on generic pharmaceuticals: a series in JAPhA. *J Am Pharm Assoc.* 2001;41:517-8.
10. Kirking DM, Ascione FJ, Gaither CA, Welage LS. Economics and structure of the generic pharmaceutical industry. *J Am Pharm Assoc.* 2001 ;41 :578-84.
11. Kirking DM, Gaither CA, Ascione FJ, Welage LS. Physicians' individual and organizational views on generic medications. *J Am Pharm Assoc.*2001;41:718 22.
12. Kirking DM, Gaither CA, Ascione FJ, Welage LS. Pharmacists' individual and organizational views on generic medications. *J Am Pharm Assoc.* 2001;41:723-8.
13. Gaither CA, Kirking DM, Ascione FJ, Welage LS. Consumers' views on generic medications. *J Am Pharm Assoc.* 2001;41:729-36.
14. Kaplan AH. Fifty years of drug amendments revisited: in easy-to-swallow capsule form. *Food Drug Law J.* 1995;50(spec iss):179-96.
15. Temin P. *Taking Your Medicine: Drug Regulation in the United States.* Cambridge, Mass: Harvard University Press; 1980;120-40.
16. Dibner MD. Biotechnology and pharmaceuticals. Ten years later. *BioPharm.* 1997;10:24-9. Cited by: WuPong S. An overview of biotechnology. In: Wu-Pong S Rojanasakul Y, eds. *Biopharmaceutical Drug Design and Development.* Totowa, NJ: Humana Press; 1999:1-19.
17. Haynes W. *The Chemical Companies.* New York, NY: D. Van Nostrand Company; 1949:469-71. *American Chemical Industry*; vol 6.
18. de Haen P. Compilations of new drugs: 1940-1975. *Pharmacy Times.* March 1976: 2-34.

Governance of Pharmacy, 1852-1902

by David B. Brushwood*

In the absence of a demonstrated need for governance, capitalist democracies generally permit open markets to provide public protection from useless or harmful products and services. Users of products and services tend to act in their own self-interest, acquiring only those products and services that are seen to be of value, and refusing to acquire products and services that are not of value. Within relatively small, isolated communities, information exchange between consumers is efficient, and the providers of less valuable products or services find themselves quickly shut out of the market. Yet, as communities expand and become more complex, and when trade between them becomes routine, information exchange between consumers becomes less efficient, and governance is required to protect consumers from useless or harmful products or services.

The mid-19th century was a watershed for the governance of American pharmacy. The size and complexity of commerce in American society had led to the prevailing view, within the rapidly organizing profession, that the time had come to centralize standard-setting for the profession. The American Pharmaceutical Association (APhA) was established in 1852, at least in part due to a recognized need to collectively fix a set of standards for the strength and quality of drugs. During the next half century, long before federal legislation directly addressed the issue, APhA worked with the United States Pharmacopeial Convention to set standards for pharmaceutical products.

It was during this second half of the 19th century that state governments began to take over from localities the responsibility for regulating the pharmacy profession. This was an important time for pharmacy, because the profession took affirmative steps during this period to separate itself from the general merchants whose products were not related to the health and welfare of consumers. Groups of pharmacists in each state worked closely with APhA, and with their state associations, to draft and pass legislation that committed

*David B. Brushwood, JD, is professor, social and administrative sciences, College of Pharmacy, University of Florida, Gainesville.

the profession to public service, and assigned responsibility for regulation of the profession to members of the profession who would serve on a state board of pharmacy. The leadership of lawyer-pharmacist James Hartley Beal was critical to the emergence of pharmacy as a self-regulating profession.

Although boards of pharmacy were not as active or as influential in the late 19th century as they are today, their very existence was significant, because they provided a framework for self-regulation of the profession, into which the federal regulation of drugs could later fit. At the close of the 19th century, there continued to be problems with drug standards and with professionalism in pharmacy practice, but the seeds had been sown for a dynamic and progressive self-regulated professional practice, with a firm commitment to public service.

The day-to-day reality of pharmacy governance during this period is perhaps best understood from a brief review of case law related to the professional practices of the time.

In July 1852, the Court of Appeals of New York reported the case of *Thomas v Winchester*,[1] in which a pharmacist had been sued for allegedly labeling extract of belladonna as extract of dandelion. The patient had been harmed by use of the former, believing it to be the latter. Contrary to what had been, until very recently, a legal tradition of *caveat emptor* (let the buyer beware), the court recognized a duty owed by the pharmacist to the patient. Observing that the business in which pharmacists engaged was different from that of ordinary merchants, the court said: "The defendant's duty arose out of the nature of his business and the danger to others incident to its mismanagement. Nothing but mischief like that which actually happened could have been expected from sending the poison falsely labeled into the market; and the defendant is justly responsible for the probable consequences of the act."

In that same year, a Kentucky court reported the case of *Fleet and Semple v Hollenkemp*.[2] In this case, the defendant pharmacist was alleged to have compounded, on prescription of a physician, a product that inadvertently contained a poisonous substance. The pharmacist was held liable, and the court explained its ruling using language that is as relevant now as it was then:

The purchasers of wines and provisions, by sight, smell and taste, may be able, without incurring any material injury, to detect their bad and unwholesome qualities; but many are wholly unable, by the taste or appearance of many drugs, to distinguish those which are poisonous from others which are innoxious, so close is their resemblance to each other; purchasers have, therefore to trust the druggist. It is upon his skill and prudence they must rely. It is, therefore, incumbent upon him that he understands his business. It is his duty to know the properties of his drugs, and to be able to distinguish them from each other. It is his duty so to qualify himself, or to employ those that are so qualified, to attend to the business of compounding and vending medicines and drugs, as that one drug may not be sold for another; and so that, when a prescription is presented to be made up, the proper medicines, and none other, be used in mixing and compounding it. As applicable to the owners of drug stores, or persons engaged in vending drugs and medicines by retail, the legal maxim should be reversed. Instead of caveat emptor, it should be caveat vendor.

This new concept of "let the seller beware" epitomized the emerging governance of pharmacy in the middle of the 19th century. Pharmacists were expected to be experts on drugs, and they were expected to process orders without error. Over the course of the next half decade, practice patterns changed and governance of practice adapted to the changes. By 1901, the Supreme Court of Iowa was sorting out the relative responsibilities of pharmacists and of the pharmacy owners who employed them. In *Burgess v Sims Drug Co.*,[3] that court considered the argument by a pharmacy that it could not be held liable for the conduct of its employee pharmacist because the pharmacist was an independently licensed professional. The pharmacist was alleged to have compounded an eye plaster that led to the patient losing his eye. Adopting a consumer expectation rationale, the court held the pharmacy liable, noting that the pharmacy had held itself out as able and willing to fill prescriptions: "It was wholly immaterial to the customer, so far as defendants' liability was concerned, whether the prescription was filled by one of the defendants or by an employee." This case emphasizes the shared responsibilities of pharmacists and their employers.

Language used in the 1902 case of *Peters v Johnson*,[4] from the Supreme Court of West Virginia, addressed two important legal expectations of the profession. First, with regard to technical accuracy in order processing, the court ruled that pharmacists "are required to be extraordinarily skillful, and to use the highest degree of care known to practical men to prevent injury." The court also ruled on the extent to which a pharmacist may be held liable for bad outcomes: "If harm may come reasonably and probably to any one from another's action, there is a duty on him so to act as to avoid such injury." These two statements appropriately summarize the previous half century of pharmacy litigation. By the beginning of the 20th century, the responsibilities of pharmacists had been fully developed as a matter of law. Pharmacists were not considered to be retail merchants; they were considered to be health care professionals with extensive duties to patients.

The high level of responsibility recognized for pharmacists, as summarized by courts of law, reflected the internal expectations developed by the profession for itself. Almost invariably, when asked to rule on a controversy brought by a patient against a pharmacist, courts during the last half of the 19th century turned to professional standards for guidance. These standards most often were found in state pharmacy acts that had been developed by pharmacists for pharmacists. It was no accident that when governance of pharmacy had the option of moving in the direction of either general merchandising or professionalism, the professional option was chosen. It was organized pharmacists who made this choice, and those who governed the profession relied on the profession's choice in determining legal responsibilities.

Perhaps the challenges of the profession seem daunting at times, because public expectations of the profession are high. It is these high expectations that create contemporary opportunities for the profession, and the genesis of these high expectations was at least in part the legal formalization of professional standards in the second half of the 19th century.

This article originally appeared in *Journal of the American Pharmaceutical Association*, 40, no. 3 (May/June 2000): 347-48.

References

1. *Thomas v Winchester*, 6 N.Y. 397 (N.Y. 1852).

2.   *Fleet and Semple v Hollenkemp*, 52 Ky. (1 B Mon.) 219 (1852).
3.   *Burgess v Sims Drug Co.*, 86 NW 307 (Iowa 1901).
4.   *Peters v Johnson*, 41 SE 190 (W.Va. 1902).

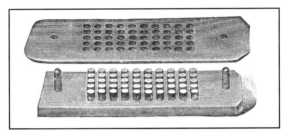

Rubber tablet mold, 1897.

Governance of Pharmacy, 1902-1952

by David B. Brushwood*

I{N} 1902 pharmacy was poised to become a dynamic and progressive patient-oriented profession. During the previous 50 years, pharmacists had firmly established themselves as health care professionals and not retail merchants. Yet, during the half-century spanning the years 1902 to 1952, governance of pharmacy shifted in focus from practice to product. The emphasis changed from enabling patients to protect themselves to protecting patients from themselves. Federal regulations became increasingly complex, resulting ultimately in centralization of decisions about drug therapy within the Food and Drug Administration (FDA) and the medical profession. Pharmacists, who at the beginning of the 20th century had helped patients make decisions about drug therapy, became dispensers of drugs to patients, who accepted them without question, relying on FDA assurances of drug safety and physician decisions about appropriate therapy.

In 1906, when the U.S. Congress passed the Pure Food and Drug Act, it would have been difficult to foresee the paternalistic approach to drug regulation that the federal authorities would take during the next 46 years. The 1906 act was based on one simple idea: Citizens who purchase foods and drugs have a right to know what they are purchasing. Patients were not forbidden to use any drugs; they were simply enabled to make better decisions for themselves by understanding what they were using.[1] By imposing requirements forbidding the adulteration or misbranding of drugs, the federal law gave consumers some measure of assurance that a drug product contained what its labeling said it contained. Consumers were then left to make their own informed decisions about product use.

The 1906 act was tested almost immediately by a manufacturer who had knowingly and falsely claimed in the labeling of its drug that the drug could cure cancer. The Supreme Court ruled that the misbranding provision of the act prevented false statements only as to a drug's identity (i.e.,

*David B. Brushwood, JD, is a pharmacist and professor of pharmacy health care administration, College of Pharmacy, University of Florida, Gainesville.

strength, quality, and purity).[2] Untruths as to other matters were not forbidden under the law. Very soon thereafter, the act was amended to prohibit "false and fraudulent" efficacy claims. This addition to the law was difficult to enforce, however, because proving fraud requires showing intent to defraud, and manufacturers could escape enforcement by claiming ignorance.

The deficiencies of the 1906 law were recognized early, yet changes to the law were slow in coming. By 1938 it had become obvious that new legislation was necessary. The catalyst for that new legislation was the "Elixir Sulfanilamide" tragedy. More than 100 patients died from using a perfectly safe drug formulated in a toxic solvent, diethylene glycol. Federal authorities were able to remove the product from the market only because its name falsely included the word "elixir," although it contained no alcohol.[3] The 1938 act, known as the Food, Drug and Cosmetic Act (FDCA), is the federal act still in force today for regulation of drug products. The most noteworthy provision of the act was the requirement that new drugs be studied for safety before they are marketed. Drugs marketed before 1938 were exempted from the act's safety requirement through a grandfather clause.

The safety assurance aspect of the 1938 act was noncontroversial. Few would argue against protecting medication users with a rule requiring studies of new drugs to determine their safety. However, a less publicized provision of the act expanded the definitions of misbranding and adulteration, resulting in a far-reaching move by the agency that should have generated controversy at the time. The misbranding provisions of the 1938 act imposed new affirmative disclosure standards for labeling, requiring inclusion of adequate directions for use and warnings about adverse effects. Under the 1906 act, a violation could occur based only on what was included in labeling, but the 1938 act recognized a violation for what was not included in labeling. The 1938 act also established an exemption under which FDA could allow drugs to be marketed without otherwise mandatory adequate directions for use and warnings if the agency determined that this labeling was not necessary for the protection of the public health. It was this exemption that eventually led to the transformation of pharmacists from drug therapy advisors to product dispensers.

Before passage of the 1938 act, patients could acquire from pharmacists any nonnarcotic drug without a prescription order. Patients who felt ill could obtain a medication order from a physician or could instead consult a pharmacist. Pharmacists could make recommendations for patients, and they could dispense a drug simply because a patient requested it. In this way, patients, physicians, and pharmacists shared responsibility for the acquisition and use of nonnarcotic drugs. In late 1938, several months after the new act took effect, FDA set in motion a series of events that would take this responsibility away from patients and pharmacists and concentrate it in the hands of physicians.

FDA interpreted the 1938 act's exemption from labeling disclosure requirements to mean that, among other conditions, if a drug was dispensed pursuant to a prescription order, then it need not be labeled with directions and warnings.[4] To be sure that a drug would be dispensed pursuant to a prescription order, FDA required that the label bear a prescription-only warning, that other warnings be directed to health care professionals, and that the drugs be shipped solely for sale pursuant to a prescription. The federal "legend" was thus born, separating so-called "legend" and "nonlegend" drugs. By permitting manufacturers to label their products, "Caution: To be used only by or on the prescription of a _____" (with the blank to be filled in with physician, dentist, or veterinarian), FDA permitted manufacturers to create a class of drugs that could not be used without a prescription.

This FDA interpretation was not discussed when Congress passed the 1938 act. It was not specifically authorized under the act, and it was taken without an opportunity for comment or compromise. Over the next several years, things began to sort themselves out with little coordinated input from pharmacists into their profession's own governance. During World War II, attentions were apparently turned to other matters. The difficulty some pharmacists faced in practice was that the labeling of pharmaceuticals determined the standard for dispensing (with or without a prescription order), and this standard was applied in different ways by different manufacturers. One manufacturer of a drug might choose to use the federal legend, while another manufacturer of the same drug might choose not to. It is hard to imagine how the most fundamental of pharmacist responsibilities could be left to the whims of a manufacturer's marketing decisions.

The chaotic situation pharmacists faced in practice was put in order by the Supreme Court in 1948. In United States v Sullivan,[5] the Court affirmed the conviction of a pharmacist who had dispensed, without a prescription order, a medication that bore the federal prescription legend when received from the manufacturer. Never mind that the same medication made by other manufacturers did not bear the legend and would not have led to a prosecution. This case established the important principle that federal law applies to the dispensing of a medication by a pharmacist to a patient within a state. It may be counterintuitive to believe that this intrastate transaction could be considered "interstate commerce" subject to federal regulation under the provisions of Article 1 of the Constitution, but the Court held that it was. The most significant aspect of this case was the court's firm recognition that FDA and the pharmaceutical manufacturers had authority to assign to physicians—at the expense of pharmacists and patients—complete responsibility for controlling patients' acquisition of the most useful medications.

The legislative reaction to this development was not what one might have expected. Rather than opposing it or seeking a compromise based on decades of responsibility over decisions about medication use, many pharmacists embraced it and sought to institutionalize it. Senator Hubert Humphrey and Congressman Carl Durham, both pharmacists, introduced legislation that would, for the first time ever, formally establish a uniform prescription-only class of drugs.[6] This legislation took effect in 1952 and led to the clear separation of dispensing pharmacists from prescribing physicians.

Why would some pharmacists be so eager to limit themselves in this way? Perhaps the answer lies in the provisions of the act regulating dispensing of refills and verbal authorization to dispense. Before 1952 it was not clear that refills could be legally authorized or that any order other than a written order was legally sufficient as a prescription. The Durham-Humphrey amendment to the FDCA clarified that refills and verbal orders were clearly permissible under the law. Apparently, the tradeoff for this concession was relinquishment of any claim of responsibility pharmacists may have had on initiation of therapy. The amendment carved out a "safe harbor" for pharmacists, who were made secure in their dispensing role but utterly excluded from primary decisions about medication use.

By 1952 pharmacists had become, through governance, what they sought to be: respected custodians of the nation's drug supply, at the tail end of the chain of distribution. This is an important role, but not a fulfillment of the promise of the profession in 1902, when an expansive patient-oriented practice appeared to be developing. Pharmacists had given over to physicians primary responsibility for making decisions about drug therapy. It would take another half-century for pharmacists to begin taking this responsibility back.

This article originally appeared in *Journal of the American Pharmaceutical Association,* 41, no. 3 (May/June 2001): 376-77.

References

1. Regier CC. The struggle for federal food and drugs legislation. *Law Contemp Prob.* 1933;1:3-15.
2. *United States v Johnson,* 221 US 488 (Sup Ct 1911).
3. Cavers DF. The Food, Drug and Cosmetic Act of 1938: its legislative history and its substantive provisions. *Law Contemp Prob.* 1939;6:2-42.
4. Temin P. The origin of compulsory drug prescription. *J Law Econ.* 1979;22:91-105.
5. *United States v Sullivan,* 332 US 689 (Sup Ct 1948).
6. Dunn CW. The new prescription drug law. *Food Drug Cosmetic Law J.* 1951; 6:951-69.

Governance of Pharmacy, 1952-2002

by David B. Brushwood*

T HE Durham-Humphrey Amendment to the Food, Drug, and Cosmetic Act, which became effective in 1952, firmly recognized pharmacists as the societally appointed dispensers of medications prepared by large-scale manufacturers and prescribed by physicians. With few exceptions, a pharmacist's responsibility at that time was limited to ensuring the accuracy of order processing. Responsibility for product integrity rested primarily with the manufacturer, and responsibility for the appropriateness of therapy rested with the physician.

As if to emphasize this limited role, in the mid-1950s states passed so-called "antisubstitution" laws, which made clear the expectation that pharmacists were to unwaveringly follow physicians' orders. Apparently, some pharmacists had not gotten the message of the federal regulation and were inappropriately substituting a different (but similar) drug in place of the drug prescribed.

By the mid-1970s the wisdom of antisubstitution laws was being questioned. Not only did these laws forbid substituting one drug for another, they also forbade substituting one brand for another brand of the same drug. If a physician prescribed a specific brand of a drug, then the pharmacist could not substitute an equally safe and effective, but less expensive, generically equivalent product. Gradually, state antisubstitution laws were repealed and replaced with product selection laws that described the circumstances and conditions under which pharmacists could select and dispense a less expensive, generically equivalent product.

The passage of product selection laws was significant for the profession because it began a shift in drug regulatory policy away from physician preeminence and back toward discretionary authority for pharmacists. This change in policy was not universally welcomed within the profession at first.[1] A 1984 amendment to the Food, Drug, and Cosmetic Act increased the availability of

---

*David B. Brushwood, JD, is a pharmacist and professor of pharmacy health care administration, College of Pharmacy, University of Florida, Gainesville.

generic products as economic pressures created incentives for the substitution of generic products for more expensive brand-name products. Generic substitution is now standard practice in the profession.

In 1970 the U.S. Congress consolidated a number of related laws regulating controlled substances, resulting in the Drug Enforcement Administration's (DEA) promulgation of regulations recognizing significant responsibilities of pharmacists. The agency's policy is that a prescription is not necessarily valid simply because it has been issued by a licensed physician with a current DEA registration.[2] To be valid, a prescription must be issued for a "legitimate medical purpose" in the "usual course of professional practice." Although the prescriber has primary responsibility for assuring a prescription's validity, the pharmacist has a "corresponding responsibility" to provide such assurance. Under this federal regulatory policy, pharmacists are required to use professional discretion in screening prescriptions for legitimacy without denying patients access to the medications necessary for their care.

Yet, even as the courts appeared to be leaning toward expanding the professional discretion of pharmacists, a single case riled the profession in a way none had before and perhaps none has since. In 1976 the U.S. Supreme Court issued its opinion in *Virginia State Board of Pharmacy v Virginia Consumer Citizens Council, Inc.*[3] The court ruled that a state board of pharmacy may not forbid the advertising of prices for pharmaceuticals because such advertising is commercial speech and is protected from government restriction under the First Amendment to the Constitution of the United States. This was the first of a series of decisions that subsequently opened up advertising by every profession. The ruling had little to do with pharmacy, but it had everything to do with free trade and the rights of consumers to make informed choices.

In a concurring opinion, Chief Justice Warren Burger initially wrote that in dispensing drugs, "The pharmacist performs three tasks: he finds the correct bottle; he counts out the correct number of tablets or measures the right amount of liquid; and he accurately transfers the doctor's dosage instructions to the container. Without minimizing the potential consequences of error in performing these tasks or the importance of the other tasks a professional pharmacist performs, it is clear that in this regard he no more renders a true professional service than does a clerk who sells lawbooks."[4] The protests from the American Pharmaceutical Association (APhA) and other representatives of the pharmacy profession were loud and long, and the pejorative language was omitted from the official opinion. Justice Burger had hit a raw nerve within the profession. The professionalism within pharmacy was not apparent to many policy makers in the mid-1970s.

Similar perceptions of pharmacists as technically competent but lacking in the skills necessary to provide direct patient care have stood in the way of the establishment of a "third class" of drugs under federal law. Pursuant to authority granted by Congress in 1962, the Food and Drug Administration had begun to switch a small number of prescription drugs to nonprescription status. Some found it illogical that a drug that had one day been considered so dangerous as to be restricted to use only under the authority of a medical doctor could on the next day be freely purchased at a grocery store or gas station. Many felt there had to be a middle ground, and pharmacists offered to facilitate prescription-to-nonprescription switches by controlling access to the drugs in question and overseeing their use on an interim basis. Suspicious that pharmacists were motivated by economics rather than professionalism, opponents contended that this was, in effect, a proposal for the creation of a "druggists' monopoly." Despite support from APhA and other pharmacy organizations, a pharmacist-controlled class of drugs has yet to be created in the United States.[5]

By 1990 federal policy makers had begun to recognize that expanded practice by pharmacists could improve drug therapy outcomes. In the Omnibus Budget Reconciliation Act of 1990 (OBRA '90), Congress established a new condition for state participation in the federally funded but state-managed Medicaid program. Under OBRA '90, states were required to promulgate standards that ensured comprehensive drug use review, including screening before dispensing and an offer of counseling by a pharmacist. Some states chose to require this program only for prescriptions written for Medicaid patients. Most states, however, through their boards of pharmacy, chose to implement this elevated standard of pharmacy practice for prescriptions dispensed to all patients.[6]

During the 1990s, state governments were active in the adoption of legislation or regulations authorizing pharmacists and physicians to enter into collaborative drug therapy management agreements.[7] APhA and state pharmacy associations emphasized the collegial and mutually beneficial aspects of such collaborations. By 2002 a majority of states had authorized collaborative drug therapy management.

In March 2002 legal opinions issued from the supreme Courts of two populous states[8, 9] underscored the metamorphosis of pharmacy practice during the previous half-century. Over the previous 4 decades, courts had been challenged to recognize expanded legal standards of pharmacy practice to include a duty to monitor drug therapy as well as a duty to warn patients of potential adverse effects. Courts had been reluctant to impose on pharmacists any legal duty beyond technical accuracy in order processing. Many courts had firmly rejected patients' allegations that pharmacists had a legal duty to protect them from harm that could be foreseen from the use of a correctly dispensed medication. By 2002 the trend seemed to be changing. Several lower courts had ruled in favor of patients whose pharmacists failed to protect them from harm, even though the pharmacists had filled the patients' prescriptions correctly.

On March 14, 2002, the Supreme Judicial Court of Massachusetts ruled in favor of a patient who alleged that his pharmacy owed him a duty to warn of the potential adverse effects of a drug dispensed to him.[8] In affirming a judgment against the defendant pharmacy for failure to warn, the court reasoned that when a patient could logically interpret warnings from a pharmacist as being a complete list of all known side effects, it was appropriate to impose on the pharmacy a duty to provide a complete list. One week later, the Supreme Court of Illinois affirmed the judgment of a lower court in favor of a patient who alleged that her pharmacy had a duty to screen her prescription for known allergies and warn either her or her physician when she was prescribed a drug to which the pharmacist knew she was allergic.[9]

Fifty years after the Durham-Humphrey Amendment became effective, pharmacists have become legally recognized as health care providers whose responsibilities include, but extend far beyond, technical accuracy in order processing. Pharmacists are legally required to evaluate drug therapy and to act appropriately so as to reduce the likelihood of bad outcomes. In collaboration with physicians, pharmacists are legally authorized to promote good outcomes from drug therapy.

Patients have a right to expect a high level of skill and care from their pharmacists. Legal standards for pharmacists reflect the high expectations patients have of pharmacists and the ability of pharmacists to meet those high expectations.

This article originally appeared in *Journal of the American Pharmaceutical Association*,42, no. 3 (May/June 2002): 383-84.

References

1. *Pharmaceutical Society of the State of New York v Lefkowitz*, 596 F2d 953 (2nd Cir 1978).
2. 21 CFR § 1306.04.
3. *Virginia State Board of Pharmacy v Virginia Consumer Citizens Council, Inc.*, 425 US 748 (1976).
4. *U.S. Law Week* May 26 1976:4686, 4693.
5. *Nonprescription Drugs. Value of a Pharmacist-Controlled Class Has Yet to Be Demonstrated*. Washington, DC: U.S. General Accounting Office: 1995. GAO-95-12.
6. Huang S. The Omnibus Reconciliation Act of 1990: redefining pharmacists' legal responsibilities. *Am J Law Med*.1998;24:417-42.
7. Ferro L, Marcrom RE, Garrelts L, et al. Collaborative practice agreements between pharmacists and physicians. *J Am Pharm Assoc*.1998;38.6556.
8. *Cottom v CVS Pharmacy* 2002 Mass. LEXIS 146 (March 14, 2002).
9. *Happel v Wal-Mart Stores Inc.*, 2002 111. LEXIS 296 (March 21, 2002).

Pharmacy Organizations, 1852-1902

by George B. Griffenhagen*

P HARMACY in the United States was organized from the top down, not from the bottom up as one might expect. There were, of course, a few local associations, most of which were represented at the founding of the American Pharmaceutical Association (APhA) in 1852; they included local pharmacy societies in Baltimore, Boston, Cincinnati, Hartford, New York City, Philadelphia, and Richmond. All but two of these associations were designated as "colleges," a term based on English custom to place pharmacy societies on the same footing as medical societies. The two 1852 local societies not designated as a college were the Connecticut group described by APhA as an "imperfect association," and the Richmond Pharmaceutical Association, whose membership was restricted to "pharmacy proprietors."[1] There was an eighth local pharmacy group in 1852 called the German Apothecary Society of New York City; it served as a social club for the German pharmacists who had immigrated to America.[2]

APhA's 1852 bylaws decreed that "every local pharmaceutical association shall be entitled to five delegates" at each annual convention, stimulating the formation of other societies, including those in Memphis, St. Louis, and Washington, D.C. By 1858, APhA corresponding secretary Edward Parrish urged pharmacists to organize a local association "in all towns which contain over eight or ten reputable pharmaceutists."[3] But there still was not a single state pharmaceutical association in the United States, and as the Civil War engulfed the nation there was a lull of nearly a decade in the formation of any pharmacy associations.

First State Associations

Two new types of pharmacy societies appeared at APhA annual conventions after the Civil War. The first, in 1865, was a delegation from the Alum-

---

*George B. Griffenhagen, retired pharmacist, is a former editor of *JAPhA*.

ni Association of the Philadelphia College of Pharmacy, which sought to be recognized as a local society to be entitled to five delegates at APhA conventions.[4] Two years later, the APhA annual meeting received word of the founding of the Maine Pharmaceutical Association; it was initially considered to be another local association, but in time this group was recognized as something quite new—the first state pharmaceutical association. Between 1871 and 1887, a total of 36 state pharmaceutical associations were organized. APhA was largely responsible for the creation of most of these, leading APhA president C. Lewis Diehl to describe the state pharmaceutical associations as "the children of APhA."[5]

Initially, state pharmaceutical associations limited their membership to pharmacy owners. For a time this restriction was of little concern to employee pharmacists, because most could eventually realize their ambition of becoming a proprietor. But by the end of the 1870s it was no longer possible for every pharmacist to achieve the goal of owning his own pharmacy. As a result, pharmacists were separated into two distinct groups. The proprietors were now known as "druggists," while employee pharmacists were designated as "drug clerks." The latter began to organize in an effort to obtain better working conditions. The first national organization for employee pharmacists was established in 1893 under the name of the Drug Clerks' Mutual Benefit Association.[6] While the druggist associations feared that these drug clerk societies could lead to unionization, APhA welcomed with open arms

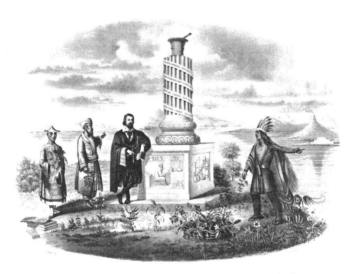

AMERICAN PHARMACEUTICAL ASSOCIATION.
FOUNDED A.D. 1852.

The first APhA membership certificate, adopted in 1855, was both ornate and symbol-laden. The central column with mortar and pestle at the top, is encircled with a scroll listing a dozen great names in pharmacy from Galen and Avicenna to Scheele and Liebig. The four figures (left to right) represent Oriental pharmacy, Arabic pharmacy, European pharmacy, and the botanicals introduced into pharmacy by Native Americans.

representatives of drug clerks' associations from Chicago, St. Louis, and Washington, D.C.

Commerical Pharmacy

While the drug clerks were seeking recognition as professional equals, the proprietors were experiencing disastrous price cutting competition from the aggressive marketing of proprietary medicines in department stores. Wholesale druggists were among the first to seek a remedy to price cutting by forming the Western Wholesale Druggists' Association in 1876. When this group became national in 1882 under the name of the National Wholesale Druggists' Association, they turned to the newly established Proprietary Association of America[a] for assistance in preventing the cutting of wholesale prices on proprietary medicines.[7] But the patent medicine manufacturers were more concerned with "the extermination of imitation goods" produced by drugstore proprietors than they were with controlling price cutting.

A growing number of pharmacy proprietors felt that APhA could no longer protect their business interests. Neither the creation of the National Retail Druggists Association at the 1883 APhA annual convention nor the establishment of APhA's Section of Commercial Interests in 1887 quelled this concern, and APhA president Henry Whitney admitted in 1898 that, "there is no national body of pharmacists that represents the commercial side of pharmacy."[8] So, on the initiative of the Chicago Retail Druggists Association, and with the encouragement of the APhA Section of Commercial Interests, the National Association of Retail Druggists (now known as the National Community Pharmacists Association) was founded in 1898.[9]

Education and Legislation

APhA was more successful in nurturing organizations of colleges of pharmacy and boards of pharmacy than they were in meeting the business needs of pharmacy proprietors. But the former efforts took a quarter century to solidify. For example, delegates from colleges of pharmacy convened at the APhA 1870 annual meeting; however, the resulting Conference of Teaching Colleges was ineffectual because the delegates were without real policy-making powers, and the conference was dissolved in 1884.[2]

APhA, which had fostered the organization of state pharmaceutical associations, did not send her children defenseless into legislative battles. The defense was a model state law to regulate the practice of pharmacy, which was drafted in 1869 by an APhA committee led by John M. Maisch, and was enacted as legislation by a number of states. The state boards of pharmacy, created by these pharmacy laws, needed knowledge and experience; therefore, APhA called for "boards to unite and form an association" in the hope that they would develop a method of reciprocity of state pharmacy licenses. Two years later, several pharmacy boards did meet with APhA, but no or-

---

[a]The Proprietary Association of America was formed in 1881 as the Association of Manufacturers and Dealers in Proprietary Articles. The Proprietary Association subsequently changed its name to the Nonprescription Drug Manufacturers Association in 1990, and then to the Consumer Health Care Products Association in 1999.

ganization was forthcoming. So, in 1889 APhA created the APhA Section on Education and Legislation to fill this void. Associations for boards of pharmacy and faculties of pharmacy came into their own at the turn of the century. The American Association of Colleges of Pharmacy was founded in 1900 as the Conference of Pharmaceutical Faculties, while the National Association of Boards of Pharmacy was established 4 years later.[5]

As APhA's semicentennial convention approached, the only other new national pharmacy associations involved recreational pursuits such as the American Drug Trade Bowling Association, founded in 1897, and the Apothecaries' Bicycle Club, founded in 1898.[6] There was a flood of new pharmacy organizations to come in the 20th century, but these will be the subject of the second and third installments in this tripartite series on the history of APhA.

This article originally appeared in *Journal of the American Pharmaceutical Association*, 40, no. 2 (March/ April 2000): 139-40.

References

1. *Proceedings of the National Pharmaceutical Convention*, October 6, 1852.
2. *The Druggists Circular*. January 1907.
3 *Proceedings of the American Pharmaceutical Association*, September 1958.
4. *Proceedings of the American Pharmaceutical Association*, 1865.
5. Sonnedecker G. *Kremers and Urdang's History of Pharmacy*. Philadelphia, Pa: Lippincott; 1976:195-8.
6. Griffenhagen G. U.S. Pharmaceutical and Related Associations, Past and Present [manuscript]. Madison, Wisc: American Institute of the History of Pharmacy; 1995.
7. Fay JT Jr. NWDA First One Hundred Years. *Wholesale Drugs*. October-November 1976.
8. *Proceedings of the American Pharmaceutical Association*, 1898.
9. Williams CF. *A Century of Service and Beyond*. NCPA, 1998.

Pharmacy Organizations, 1902-1952

*by George B. Griffenhagen**

T HE first half of the 20th century was a time of increasing specialization in the pharmacy profession. This article reviews how new developments in the profession during that period were reflected in changes in APhA's organizational structure, changes that on occasion led to the birth of other pharmacy organizations.

In 1900 APhA had a total membership of 1,263, which consisted mainly of practicing pharmacists (who were still called "druggists"), professors at 34 schools of pharmacy, and representatives of more than two dozen drug manufacturers and wholesalers. There were few employee pharmacists (then considered "drug clerks") and even fewer women. Those members who attended the APhA Annual Meeting in 1900 were able to present contributed papers before four different Sections, all of which were created in 1887 "to expedite and render more efficient the work of the Association."

Scientific Section

Scientific presentations were delegated to the Scientific Section, and were mainly devoted to the identity, standardization, and use of such drugs as belladonna, cannabis, cascara sagrada, cod liver oil, digitalis, ergot, ipecac, opium, pepsin, quinine, and strychnine.

As evidence of the section's activity, more than 2,500 different papers were presented before the Scientific Section from 1887 to 1952. The Scientific Section survived under its original name throughout the entire first half of the 20th century.[1]

Section on Commercial Interests

Charged to find a way to "protect the business interests of its members,"

---

*George B. Griffenhagen, retired pharmacist, is a former editor of *JAPhA*.

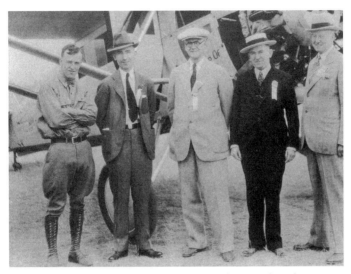

Closer relations between APhA and NARD were discussed as the two associa-
tion presidents flew over Mt. Rushmore during the APhA 1929 Annual Meeting
in Rapid City, South Dakota. The group includes (left to right) pilot Ed Hefley;
APhA secretary Evander F. Kelly; APhA president David F. Jones; NARD presi-
dent Denny Brown; and APhA local secretary Floyd W. Brown.

the Section on Commercial Interests faced more complex issues. Competition in the sale of proprietary medicines had become an integral part of pharmacy. Traditional pharmacies were failing as a result of the demoralizing trend of "price cutting," or selling the proprietary medicines for less than the usual resale price established by the manufacturer. Significantly, many of the most successful cut-rate drugstores were operated by enterprising nonpharmacist businessmen.

After trying without success to remedy the situation, Joseph Price Remington told the Section members in 1895 that, "there is a need for the retail druggists to get together and form an organization in which they will not admit the wholesaler, the professor in the college of pharmacy, or the proprietor of a remedy; but a retail druggists association pure and simply which shall be controlled by the retail druggists of this country."

Remington's exhortation led to the formation in 1898 of the first specialty organization for pharmacy practitioners, the National Association of Retail Druggists. The following year APhA president Charles Emile Dohme told the APhA convention that "NARD has sprung into existence since our last meeting and is actively engaged in the very laudable attempt to eliminate the much dreaded and despised cut-rate evil. I sincerely hope the NARD will succeed in its efforts."

To establish closer ties, NARD president Henry P. Hynson was elected chairman *pro tem* of the 1899 APhA Commercial Section. In 1901 NARD president William C. Anderson addressed the Commercial Section, anticipating the day when "these two organizations, standing shoulder to shoulder, shall form the firm foundation on which is built the magnificent structure, American pharmacy." One year later, NARD executive secretary Thomas

Wooten was elected chairman of the Commercial Section, and told the group, "You are charged—unjustly I know—with being out of touch with the man behind the prescription counter. If pharmacy is to continue to be a remunerative calling, the commercial side of pharmacy always must have a champion."

APhA proposed in 1902 that NARD and APhA hold a joint convention, but no mutually acceptable location and date could be found. This marked the beginning of a slow decline in relations between NARD and the APhA Commercial Section, as the two organizations thereafter could find few points of agreement. Recognizing that this fractious situation was working against the interests of practitioners, in 1905 APhA president Joseph Lemberger suggested that the Commercial Section be disbanded. Nevertheless, the Section remained intact until 1937, when its name was changed to the Section on Pharmaceutical Economics to encompass the expanding role of economics, social, and administrative sciences that were being taught in the schools of pharmacy.

Section on Pharmaceutical Education and Legislation

The inability of the schools of pharmacy to form their own specialized organization led to the establishment of the APhA Section on Pharmaceutical Education.[2] In April 1900 the officers of the Section on Pharmaceutical Education sent a circular letter to "all the institutions in the U.S. teaching pharmacy," inviting each to send three delegates to the 1900 APhA convention in Richmond, Virginia. The American Conference on Pharmaceutical Faculties, precursor of the American Association of Colleges of Pharmacy, was thus formed on May 9, 1900, at the APhA Annual Meeting.[3]

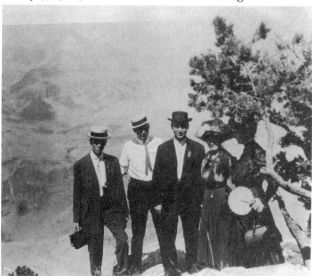

Delegates to the 1912 APhA Annual Meeting in Denver, Colorado, stop to pose by the Grand Canyon. It was on the long train trip to Denver that general secreatary James Beal and treasurer Henry Whelpley drew up the blue print for the creation of the APhA House of Delegates.

Soon after its formation in 1887, the APhA Section on Pharmaceutical Legislation surveyed state boards to determine the possibility of reciprocation of state pharmacy licenses. On the basis of the favorable responses, the Section passed a resolution asking APhA to "draw up a general plan for the interchange of certificates of the different Boards."

In the absence of any concrete action by the state boards of pharmacy, long-time APhA treasurer Henry M. Whelpley urged the APhA Section on Education and Legislation in 1903 to form a sub-section called "Conference of Board of Pharmacy Members," to begin in 1904. A motion was adopted, and a committee of five was appointed to arrange for the conference.

The result was the birth of another specialized organization. The National Association of Boards of Pharmacy was established at the 1904 APhA Annual Convention in Kansas City, and the following year they appointed a committee to prepare a constitution and bylaws for approval at the APhA Annual Meeting in Atlantic City. According to Melvin Green, "since both the Conference of Pharmaceutical Faculties and the National Association of Boards of Pharmacy were children of the APhA Sections on Education and Legislation, and since their creations were separated by only four years, it is not surprising that the two organizations met at each APhA annual meeting for many years, and their proceedings were published as part of the APhA Proceedings for more than two dozen years."[4]

The American Council on Pharmaceutical Education was founded in 1932 as a direct outgrowth of a committee created by NABP 5 years earlier. The American Foundation for Pharmaceutical Education was founded in 1942 to guarantee financial support to many colleges during World War II; subsequently the Foundation supported the Pharmaceutical Survey, whose launching in 1946 by Edward C. Elliott was a milestone in the history of American pharmacy.

Organizations for Practitioners

During the first half of the 20th century, only three new APhA Sections were created. The Section on Practical Pharmacy and Dispensing was formed in 1900 as an exclusive organization for practicing pharmacists. Henry Vincome Arny (who was to become APhA 1923-1924 president) presented a paper before the Section in 1914 recommending that, "practicing prescriptionists of this association form an organization called the American Institute of Prescriptionists" to provide a special forum for the increasing number of exclusive prescription pharmacists. But it was not until 1940 that this goal was realized with the establishment of the American College of Apothecaries.[5]

Hospital Pharmacists

As early as 1921, APhA president Charles Herbert Packard pointed out that "there are in the whole country over 6,000 hospitals; probably over 500 of these employ pharmacists." He therefore recommended that a hospital pharmacists' committee be created and given a part in the program of the APhA Section on Practical Pharmacy and Dispensing. In 1922 all of the Section officers were hospital pharmacists, a circumstance that no doubt influenced the Section's proposal that a separate section for hospital pharmacists be organized.

For the remainder of the 1920s, there was a leveling off in hospital pharmacy organizational efforts, but articles on hospital pharmacy still appeared in almost every issue of JAPhA from 1926 through 1935. In 1936 a group of 10 hospital pharmacists persuaded Association officials at that year's APhA Annual Meeting to establish a subsection on hospital pharmacy within the Section on Practical Pharmacy and Dispensing. J. Solon Modell, one of the early leaders of the hospital pharmacy movement, described this action as "a turning point and milestone in the development of hospital pharmacy practice."

Still, it was not enough. In 1940 the APhA House of Delegates expressed "a real need for a unified organization of hospital pharmacists." In 1941 the House approved a resolution that the APhA sub-section on hospital pharmacy should be abolished and a new specialized group formed. On August 21, 1942, the new organization, American Society of Hospital Pharmacists, was approved by the APhA Council as an APhA affiliate. The sub-section was dissolved, and the inaugural meeting of ASHP was held at the 1943 APhA Annual Meeting with Harvey A. K. Whitney as the first president. ASHP changed its name in 1994 to the American Society of Health-System Pharmacists to expand its membership base.

Employee Pharmacists

By the late 19th century, employee pharmacists (still called "drug clerks") had begun to organize in an effort to obtain better working conditions, viewing their working hours as too long and their salaries as insufficient. Whereas state pharmaceutical associations restricted their membership to pharmacy owners, APhA welcomed with open arms representatives of these drug clerks' associations. The first national organization for employee pharmacists was the Drug Clerks' Mutual Benefit Association, established in 1893. Other organizations of employee pharmacists created in the early 20th century included the American Registered Pharmacists Association, founded in 1900, and the Drug Clerks' Brotherhood, founded in 1908. The National Drug Clerks Association operated a home for "aged and infirm drug clerks" from 1924 until the group was dissolved in 1934.

Two other specialty organizations were formed in the first half of the 20th century. State pharmaceutical associations created the National Council of State Pharmaceutical Association Executives (NCSPAE) in 1927 as the Conference of Pharmaceutical Association Secretaries. Local pharmacy societies established the Metropolitan Pharmaceutical Association Secretaries the following year (1928).

Chain Pharmacies

Before 1890, few pharmacists owned and operated two or more pharmacies. Ten years later, in 1900, there were no more than 25 pharmacies in the country that could be called chains. But by 1920 chain pharmacies were flourishing, with a total of 1,565 chain pharmacies representing 3% of all drugstores in the United States. The largest were the Louis K. Liggett Company (New York City) with 211 pharmacies, the Owl Drug Company (San Francisco) with 32 pharmacies, and the Walgreen Drug Company (Chicago) with 21 pharmacies.

The National Association of Chain Drugstores (NACDS) was organized in 1933 by Wallace J. Smith of Read Drug and Chemical Co. (now Rite Aid) to establish "a unified voice to represent chains for the 1933 Retail Drug Code Authority."

APhA House of Delegates

Perhaps the most important organizational action of APhA in the first half of the 20th century was the creation of the House of Delegates. The idea first arose on the long train trip to Denver for the 1912 APhA Annual Meeting when APhA general secretary James Hartley Beal and long-time APhA treasurer Henry M. Whelpley discussed the need for a body within APhA that could represent the thinking of all of the specialties within the profession. After a spirited debate in Denver, the APhA House of Delegates was formally organized on August 21, 1912. Two days earlier the APhA Council (now the Board of Trustees) had adopted an enabling resolution charging the new body "to receive and consider the reports of delegates from the bodies they represent."

The APhA House of Delegates was not an immediate success. Evander F. Kelly (who later became APhA chief executive officer) concluded in his address as 1921 chairman of the House that "the House has not fulfilled the expectations of those who established it." Kelly urged the House "to take proper steps to see that the state associations, as the basic units of the House, shall have the opportunity to express themselves concerning its [APhA's] organization, and how they may be brought into the originally intended relation to APhA."

The House of Delegates promptly adopted a resolution urging the APhA Council to support the House with the necessary financial aid and to seek "every available means to bring state pharmaceutical associations into active participation in the House." By 1923 a reorganization plan had been developed, 23 state associations had affiliated, all of them were qualified to send voting delegates to the House.

The day following the creation of the APhA House of Delegates, the APhA Council adopted another resolution, this one recommending the creation of a body consisting of delegates of the then-existing national drug and pharmaceutical associations. The Council envisioned that this new body would consider legislation relating to both the production and distribution of drugs as well as the professional practice of pharmacy. Thus the National Drug Trade Conference was established on January 15, 1913. APhA Section of Legislation and Education chairman John Crawford Wallace served as the first president from 1913 to 1918. The name of the group was changed in 1996 to the National Conference of Pharmaceutical Organizations.

Pharmaceutical Industry

The first half of the 20th century saw a proliferation of associations of pharmaceutical manufacturers. The Nonprescription Drug Manufacturers Association (NDMA), which changed its name in 1898 from the Association of Manufacturers and Dealers in Proprietary Articles, was the only major association representing the pharmaceutical industry at the turn of the century. The American Association of Pharmaceutical Chemists was founded in 1907, and the National Association of Manufacturers of Medicinal Products was organized in 1912. It was not until 1958 that these organizations merged to form the Pharmaceutical Manufacturers Association, now known as the Pharmaceutical Research and Manufacturers of America.[8] The Parenteral Drug Association was founded in 1946.

Pharmaceutical Wholesalers

The only association of pharmaceutical wholesalers in 1900 was the National Wholesale Druggists Association, which had been founded in 1876 as the Western Wholesale Druggists Association.[9] By 1900 there were 662 wholesale druggists (pharmacies that sold both retail and wholesale prices) and 200 exclusive pharmaceutical wholesalers servicing 28,000 pharmacies.

Believing they could save money by grouping their purchases from wholesalers and manufacturers, many pharmacists participated in "buying clubs." By 1905 so many "buying clubs" were operating that they organized as the American Druggists Syndicate that year, and as the Associated Drug Companies of America in 1906. Both associations were succeeded by the Federal Wholesale Druggists' Association (FWDA) in 1915. For years FWDA limited its membership to these "buying clubs," now termed as "pharmacy-owned cooperatives," but in 1940 the Association opened its membership to other exclusive wholesalers. In the second half of the 20th century FWDA and other wholesalers associations merged with the National Wholesalers

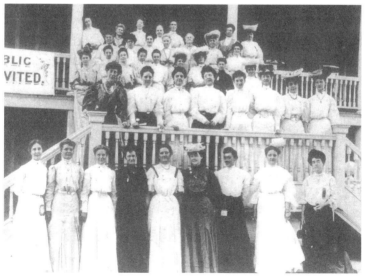

Wives of APhA members, and the few women pharmacist-members who were in attendance, gather at the 1905 APhA Annual Meeting in Atlantic City, N J. They chose to call themselves the "Women's Auxiliary." The APhA Women's Section was created 7 years later. The APhA Auxiliary, officially established in 1936, included both male and female spouses of members.

Druggists Association (NWDA). In January 2001 NWDA changed its name to the Healthcare Distribution Management Association.

Women's Organizations

In 1900 only 2% of pharmacy students were women. Even so, an independent Woman's Pharmaceutical Association already existed, having been formed in 1892 for Illinois women pharmacists; it became national in 1903 with 16 chapters. This was followed in 1905 by the Pacific Coast Woman's Pharmaceutical Association.

An APhA Women's Section was founded in 1912 to "emphasize the right and capability of women to engage in pharmaceutical pursuits [and] to unite the women members of APhA." However, the Women's Section dissolved 11 years later, as were other women's pharmaceutical associations, to encourage women to join men's organizations. The APhA Women's Auxiliary was established in 1936 for the spouses of APhA members; the name was changed in 1978 to the APhA Auxiliary to accommodate members' male spouses.

The only other new APhA Section created during the first half of the 20th century was the Section on Historical Pharmacy, established in 1902. This Section subsequently merged with the American Institute of the History of Pharmacy, which was founded in 1941 and still meets annually at APhA annual meetings.

Fraternities

Specialized pharmacy fraternities came into being during the first half of the 20th century. Before this, pharmacists seeking fellowship were limited to the Kappa Psi Pharmaceutical Fraternity, which was founded in 1879 as a medical fraternity, but opened its membership to pharmacists in 1897. Phi Delta Chi Pharmaceutical Fraternity was founded as the Phi Chi Society in 1883, but changed their name to Phi Delta Chi in 1909 to avoid to confusion with Phi Chi Medical Fraternity.

Pharmacy fraternities that came into their own between 1902 and 1952 included Alpha Zeta Omega Pharmaceutical Fraternity (AZO) in 1919; Rho Pi Phi Pharmaceutical Fraternity in 1922; and Rho Chi Honor Society in 1922, when Aristolochite Society, created in 1908 at the University of Michigan, became national. Pharmaceutical sororities include Lambda Kappa Sigma Pharmaceutical Sorority which was founded in 1913 at Massachusetts College of Pharmacy, and became national in 1918; and Kappa Epsilon Pharmaceutical Sorority was founded in 1921.

The trend toward increasing specialization of pharmacy organizations persisted through the second half of the 20th century, which will be covered in the third and final installment of Pharmacy Organizations in the APhA Sesquicentennial series.

This article originally appeared in *Journal of the American Pharmaceutical Association*, 41, no. 2 (March/April 2001): 166-70.

References

1. Griffenhagen G. The scientific section of the American Pharmaceutical Association. *Am J Pharm Ed.* 1953;17:342-50.
2. Sonnedecker G. The section on education and legislation of the American Pharmaceutical Association. *Am J Pharm Ed.* 1953;17:362-83.
3. Buerki RA. The first century of the American Association of Colleges of Pharmacy. *Am J Pharm Ed.* 1999;63(suppl):210.
4. Green MW. *The First 75 Years of the National Association of Boards of Pharmacy.* Chicago, Ill: National Association of Boards of Pharmacy; 1979.
5. Stieb EW. *First Quarter Century of the American College of Apothecaries.* Bartlett, Tenn.: ACA; 1970.
6. Harris RR, McConnell WE. The American Society of Hospital Pharmacists: a history. *Am J Hosp Pharm.* 1993; 6(suppl 2).
7. Cope JD. *The Story of the National Conference of Pharmaceutical Organizations.* Washington, D.C.:1996.
8. Cray WC. *The First 30 Years: The Pharmaceutical Manufacturers Association.* Washington, D.C.: Pharmaceutical Manufacturers Association; 1989.
9. Fay JT Jr. *NWDA First One Hundred Years 1876-1976.* Indianapolis, Ind.; 1976.

Pharmacy Organizations, 1952-2002

*by George B. Griffenhagen**

T HE primary organizations of pharmacy were already in place in 1952. The APhA Council, whose name was changed to APhA Board of Trustees in 1966, was formed in 1880, and the APhA House of Delegates was created in 1912.[1] One of the by-products of the 1952 APhA centennial meeting was the incorporation of the APhA Foundation[2] on May 6, 1953.

In 1952 APhA had five Sections: the Scientific Section and the Pharmaceutical and Education Section, both created in 1887; the Practical Pharmacy Section, formed in 1900; the Historical Pharmacy Section, which existed from 1902 until it merged with the American Institute of the History of Pharmacy (AIHP)[3] in 1968; and the Pharmaceutical Economics Section, which formed in 1937 and replaced the Commercial Interests Section founded in 1887.[1]

Other national pharmacy associations operating in 1952 included the following:

- National Association of Retail Druggists, founded in 1898; the organization changed its name in 1996 to the National Community Pharmacists Association.[4]
- American Association of Colleges of Pharmacy, founded in 1900 as the Conference of Pharmaceutical Faculties.[5]
- National Association of Boards of Pharmacy, founded in 1904.[6]
- American Council on Pharmaceutical Education, founded in 1932.[7]
- National Association of Chain Drug Stores, founded in 1933.[8]
- American College of Apothecaries, founded in 1940.[9]
- American Society of Hospital Pharmacists, founded in 1942; the organization changed its name in 1994 to the American Society of Health-System Pharmacists (ASHP).[10]
- American Foundation for Pharmaceutical Education, founded in 1942.[11]
- National Pharmaceutical Association, founded in 1949.[1]

---

*George B. Griffenhagen, retired pharmacist, is a former editor of *JAPhA*.

Pharmaceutical industry associations that existed in 1952 included the following:

• National Wholesale Druggists Association, which was established in 1876 as the Western Wholesale Druggists Association and changed its name again in 2001 to Healthcare Distribution Management Association.[12]

• Proprietary Association, founded in 1881, which changed its name to the Nonprescription Drug Manufacturers Association in 1990 and then to the Consumer Healthcare Products Association in 1999.[13]

• American Drug Manufacturers Association, founded in 1907, and American Drug Manufacturers Association, founded in 1912.[14] These organizations merged in 1958 to become the Pharmaceutical Manufacturers Association,[15] which changed its name in 1994 to Pharmaceutical Research and Manufacturers of America.

• Parenteral Drug Association, founded in 1946.[1]

In 1952 the National Drug Trade Conference, organized in 1913 by APhA, also operated. This organization was composed of the chief executive officers of industry and pharmacy associations.[16] As its membership expanded, the organization was renamed in 1996 as the National Conference of Pharmaceutical Organizations.[17] However, it was not until 1977 that a similar organization limited to the representatives of national professional pharmacy organizations was formed, the Joint Commission of Pharmacy Practitioners.[1]

APhA Sections and Academies

To meet the challenges practicing pharmacists faced as their professional responsibilities expanded, APhA established the Section on General Practice of Pharmacy in 1961.[18] To accommodate pharmacists in industry, the Industrial Pharmacy Section was formed in 1959, followed by the Pharmaceutical Technology Section in 1961. Finally, in 1965, APhA merged most existing sections into two Academies: the Academy of General Practice of Pharmacy and the Academy of Pharmaceutical Sciences (APS). The former included the Section on General Practice of Pharmacy and the Economics and Administrative Science Section. The Military Section, created in 1956, and having changed its name in 1973 to the Federal Pharmacy Section, remained intact until 1990, when it was dissolved.

APS[19] created a variety of new sections:

• Basic Pharmaceutics (the core of the former Scientific Section).

• Drug Standards, Analysis and Control (renamed Pharmaceutical Analysis and Control in 1969).

• Industrial Pharmaceutical Technology (a merger of the former Industrial Pharmacy and Pharmaceutical Technology Sections).

• Medicinal Chemistry.

• Pharmacognosy and Natural Products (merging with Medicinal Chemistry in 1979).

• Pharmacology and Biochemistry (renamed Pharmacology and Toxicology in 1972).

To further strengthen its organizational structure for practicing phar-

macists, APhA created the Section of Practice Management in 1978, which became the Academy of Pharmaceutical Management in 1985. This short-lived Academy merged in 1987 with the Academy of General Practice of Pharmacy to form the Academy of Pharmacy Practice and Management (APhA-APPM). The Academy comprises the following sections:
• Administrative Practice.
• Clinical/Pharmacotherapeutic Practice (which had existed as the Clinical Practice Section since 1974).
• Community and Ambulatory Practice.
• Hospital and Institutional Practice.
• Nuclear Pharmacy Practice (which had existed since 1975)[20]
• Specialized Pharmaceutical Services.

Sections that were initially included in APhA-APPM, but replaced 2 years later to avoid duplication, were Long-term Care (established in 1975) and Home Health Care (created in 1984).[1]

Pharmaceutical Scientists

After World War II, the growth of the pharmaceutical sciences exploded. The "new breed" of pharmaceutical scientists began to feel that they were not being adequately represented within the framework of APhA. Many members of APS felt that the participation of pharmaceutical scientists who were not pharmacists was essential to the Academy's viability as an organization. Thus, a new category of APhA membership was created in 1966, that of Scientific Associate. Such members were pharmaceutical scientists who were not pharmacists and did not have full rights to vote or hold office in the parent organization. These restrictions led many members in the Scientific Associate category to consider themselves second-class citizens.

Another major concern that intensified the Academy's conflict with its parent body was whether APS could adopt a policy position that directly conflicted with APhA policy. The prime example was APhA's 1971 *White Paper on the Pharmacist's Role in Drug Product Selection*.[21] In its 1985 strategic plan, APS concluded that the Academy "should enjoy a high degree of autonomy within the framework of APhA, essentially managing its own affairs and publications." Crucial to this autonomy, APS contended, was maintaining "operational control of the *Journal of Pharmaceutical Sciences*," which APhA was not willing to grant.

In an effort to avert a threatened APS withdrawal from the Association, APhA appointed a task force to "investigate both the needs of pharmaceutical scientists and the scientific needs of APhA, and to seek such structural organizational arrangements that will accommodate the needs of both groups." The task force recommended that "the new Academy of Pharmaceutical Sciences [should] be an organization financially and administratively independent, yet have a strong collaborative relationship with APhA in areas of common interests."[1] But the window of opportunity for reconciliation had passed, and APS's officers resigned at the March 1986 APhA Annual Meeting and immediately formed their own association called the American Association of Pharmaceutical Scientists (AAPS). In 1987 APhA changed its own science Academy's name to the Academy of Pharmaceutical Research and Science

(APhA-APRS)[22] to avoid confusion with the new AAPS and to indicate that the science initiative remained an integral part of APhA. New Sections were created for Economic, Social and Administrative Sciences and Clinical Sciences. In 2001 APhA and AAPS entered into an agreement to collaborate on activities of mutual benefit to both organizations.[1]

Pharmacy Students

Recognizing the need for an official student forum, the APhA House of Delegates in 1952 recommended the establishment of a Section for Pharmacy Students. Thus, the APhA Student Section was founded in 1954. APhA then upgraded the Student Section to the Student American Pharmaceutical Association in 1969, which was known as Student APhA from 1969 to 1972, and SAPhA from 1972 to 1983, during which time students established their own House of Delegates. In 1986 SAPhA became the APhA Academy of Students of Pharmacy (APhA-ASP), gaining 25 delegates to the APhA House of Delegates.

In 1997 the pharmacy students in the organization achieved a goal they had sought since the 1970s—a seat on the APhA Board of Trustees. This was done by way of an amendment of the APhA Bylaws making all three Academy presidents voting members of the APhA Board of Trustees.[23]

The Student National Pharmaceutical Association (SNPhA) was founded in 1972 as an affiliate of the National Pharmaceutical Association. This organization is dedicated to representing the views and ideals of minority pharmacists on critical issues affecting health care and pharmacy. In recent years APhA-ASP and SNPhA have co-sponsored various health related programs.[1]

Pharmacy Technicians

Prior to 1980 APhA endorsed the use of the term "pharmacy aide" to designate support personnel utilized in pharmacy practice and advocated the training of these pharmacy aides "via in-service or on-the-job training programs." Then, in 1988, APhA officially changed the terminology to "pharmacy technician," and the Michigan Pharmacists Association (MPA) began to administer voluntary certification examinations for pharmacy technicians. The Illinois Council of Hospital Pharmacists (ICHP) followed suit. In 1993 APhA, ASHP, MPA, and ICHP agreed to develop a national voluntary certification program for technicians. In January 1995 the Pharmacy Technician Certification Board was formed to administer a voluntary test three times a year at more than 120 sites across the country. A technician who passes the examination is designated as a Certified Pharmacy Technician, and more than 100,000 pharmacy technicians have been certified to date.[1,24]

Clinical Pharmacy Emerges

As early as 1922, John C. Krantz Jr. urged that "clinical services must be a phase of pharmaceutical service." The mature concept of clinical pharmacy was first put forward in 1945 by L. Wait Rising, and Glenn Sperandio pointed out in 1965 that clinical pharmacy must include both community and hospital pharmacy. ASHP and APhA developed a definition of clinical pharmacy in 1968 that included the key phrase "patient-oriented practice."[1] The APhA Clinical Practice Section was established in 1975 to support clinical pharmacy services in all practice settings and to provide Section members with the necessary tools to advance pharmacy practice.

The American College of Clinical Pharmacy (ACCP)[25] was founded in 1979 as a professional and scientific society providing advocacy and resources enabling clinical pharmacists to achieve excellence in practice. In 1984 ACCP submitted a petition to the Board of Pharmaceutical Specialties (BPS) requesting recognition of clinical pharmacy as a specialty. BPS, however, rejected the petition in 1985, contending "clinical pharmacy practice is too broad and too general to be recognized as a specialty." ACCP crafted a new petition that more narrowly defined the tasks and skills of a clinical pharmacist, and gave the new specialty the name "pharmacotherapy." In 1988 BPS approved this petition. Today, ACCP includes both "clinical pharmacy" and "patient pharmacotherapy" in its mission statement, while the name of the APhA Clinical Practice Section was changed to Clinical/Pharmacotherapeutic Practice Section in 1987.

Even as the definition of clinical pharmacy was being debated, the American Society of Consultant Pharmacists (ASCP)[26] was founded in 1969 to assist consultant pharmacists in their role as medication experts working to ensure that their patients' medications are appropriate, effective, safe, and used correctly. Today, ASCP devotes most of its attention to senior care pharmacy in nursing facilities, psychiatric hospitals, hospice programs, and home- and community-based care.

Board of Pharmaceutical Specialties

With the development of specialties in pharmacy practice, the APhA House of Delegates in 1971 urged the creation of "an organizational mechanism within the structure of APhA for recognition of specialties and certification of specialists."[1] A task force was created in January 1973, and among their 1974 recommendations was the establishment of BPS.

BPS[27] came into existence on January 5, 1976, and promptly established criteria for the recognition of certain specialties. On June 19, 1978, BPS recognized nuclear pharmacy as the first pharmacy specialty, a step that had been encouraged by the establishment of the APhA Section on Nuclear Pharmacy 3 years earlier.[27]

In addition to pharmacotherapy (previously mentioned), BPS approved nutritional support pharmacy as a specialty in 1988, psychotherapy in 1992, and oncology pharmacy in 1996. By January 2000 nearly 3,000 pharmacists distributed across the five specialties held BPS certifications.

Managed Care

Managed health care delivery systems blossomed during the 1980s. The Academy of Managed Care Pharmacy (AMCP) was founded in 1989 as a professional society serving the needs of pharmacists working in managed care.[28]

Another national organization for managed care pharmacy can trace its origin to the introduction of a new delivery system for prescription medication. In December 1959 Ethel Percy Andrus, president of the American Association of Retired Persons, explained how her organization had instituted a prescription mail order service. She presented this testimony in hearings before the Senate Judiciary Committee's Subcommittee on Antitrust and Monopoly chaired by Estes Kefauver (D-Tenn.).

Immediately following this disclosure, all national pharmacy associations determined that "this new mechanism is enveloping and imposing a threat to pharmaceutical service.'" However, by 1975 there were enough mail order prescription firms in existence to justify the formation of the National Association of Mail Order Pharmacists. The organization's name was changed to American Managed Care Pharmacy Association in 1989 and to Pharmaceutical Care Management Association (PCMA) in 1996.[29] PCMA now represents third party administrators, health insurance companies, drug wholesalers, pharmaceutical manufacturers, and community pharmacy networks.

Pharmaceutical Care

The term "pharmaceutical care" was first used in the literature in 1954 to describe the pharmacist's interaction with the patient. Charles D. Hepler began to use the term in the 1980s to emphasize pharmacy's role as a clinical profession. Then, in 1990, Linda Strand and Hepler defined pharmaceutical care as a practice in which pharmacists assumed responsibility for their patients' drug therapy by making decisions and playing an active role in ensuring the appropriateness of therapy.[1]

Many significant joint organizational efforts were undertaken to advance the pharmaceutical care philosophy. As early as 1989, the American Association of Colleges of Pharmacy recognized that a comprehensive curriculum was required to prepare pharmacists to provide pharmaceutical care. In 1994 APhA formulated the *Principles of Practice for Pharmaceutical Care* (see www.aphanet.org/pharmcare/prinprac.html), and the APhA Foundation launched a new periodical, *Pharmaceutical Care Profiles*, published the first *Pharmaceutical Care Networking Directory*, and awarded the first grants to help pharmacists design and implement pharmaceutical care programs. "Concept Pharmacy," developed by APhA and the National Wholesale Druggists Association to demonstrate pharmaceutical care in action, premiered at the 1996 APhA Annual Meeting in Nashville, Tenn. Two years later, ASHP updated its *Clinical Skills* series to identify 10 functions of pharmaceutical care; the series provided details on implementing each of those functions in practice. In 2001 APhA and AIHP co-sponsored a symposium titled "Decade of Pharmaceutical Care."[30]

Other Organizations

Organizations formed since 1952, other than those previously mentioned, include the following:[1]

- National Pharmaceutical Council, founded in 1953 as a trade association conducting public relations for the major research-oriented pharmaceutical manufacturers.
- Pharmaceutical Distributors International, founded in 1956 as the Pharma-

ceutical Wholesalers Association and absorbed in 1984 by the Healthcare Distribution Management Association.
• American Society of Pharmacognosy, founded in 1959 as an outgrowth of the Plant Science Seminar, formed in 1923.
• Drug Information Association, founded in 1965.
• American Society for Pharmacy Law, formed in 1974 by 17 pharmacist-lawyers (the society meets every year at the APhA Annual Meeting).
• International Pharmaceutical Distributors Association, established in 1974 by merger of the Pharmaceutical Distributors International and the Federal Wholesale Druggists' Association formed in 1915, then absorbed in 1984 by the Healthcare Distribution Management Association.
• National Council on Patient Information and Education, founded in 1982 as a nonprofit coalition of over 150 organizations with the goal of improving communication of information on the appropriate use of medications to consumers and health care professionals.
• Christian Pharmacists Fellowship International, founded in 1984 as a worldwide nondenominational association of pharmacists working in all areas of pharmaceutical service.
• Generic Pharmaceutical Association, created in 2001 by the merger of the National Association of Pharmaceutical Manufacturers, founded in 1955, and the Generic Pharmaceutical Industry Association, founded in 1981.

Thus, pharmacy entered the 21st century with an amazing variety of pharmaceutical organizations reflecting both the growth and diversity of the profession.

This article originally appeared in *Journal of the American Pharmaceutical Association,* 42, no. 2 (March/April 2002): 164-68.

References

1. Griffenhagen G, Higby GJ, Sonnedecker G, Swann J eds. *150 Years of Caring: A Pictorial History of the American Pharmaceutical Association.* Washington, DC: American Pharmaceutical Association; 2002.
2. *American Pharmaceutical Association Foundation.* Washington, DC: American Pharmaceutical Association Foundation: 1990.
3. Stieb EW. *American Institute of the History of Pharmacy Through Two Decades.* Madison, Wis: American Institute of the History of Pharmacy.
4. Williams CF. *A Century of Service and Beyond: 1898 NAPD/1998 NCPA: A History of One Hundred Years of Leadership for Independent Pharmacy.* Alexandria, Va: National Community Pharmacists Association; 1998.
5. Buerki RA. The first century of the American Association of Colleges of Pharmacy. *Am J Pharm Educ.* 1999;63(suppl): 1-210.
6. Green MW. *The First 75 Years of the National Association of Boards of Pharmacy.* Chicago, Ill: National Association of Boards of Pharmacy; 1979.
7. Swain RL. A.C.P.E. conceived. *J Am Pharm Assoc* (Pract Pharm Ed). 1954;15:484 5.
8. Mobley J. *Prescription for Success: The Chain Drug Story.* Kansas City, Mo: Hallmark Cards, Lowell Press; 1990.
9. Stieb EW. *First Quarter Century of the American College of Apothecaries.* American College of Apothecaries; 1970.
10. Harris RR, McConnell WE. The American Society of Hospital Pharmacists: a history. *Am J Hosp Pharm.* 1993;50(6 suppl 2):S3 45.

11. Fischer AB Jr. *A Half-Century of Service to Pharmacy, 1942-1992*. Rockville, Md: American Foundation for Pharmaceutical Education; 1992.

12. Fay JT Jr. *Managing Healthcare Distribution, 1876-2001*. Lakewood, Colo: E.L.F. Publications; 2001.

13. Kemp EF. Some notes on the history of the Proprietary Association. *J Am Pharm Assoc*. 1926;15:973 9.

14. Maltbie BL. *A Quarter Century of Progress in Manufacturing Pharmacy*. New York, NY: American Pharmaceutical Manufacturers Association; 1937.

15. Cray WC. *The First 30 Years The Pharmaceutical Manufacturers Association*. Washington, DC: Pharmaceutical Manufacturers Association; 1989.

16. Cope JD. *The Story of the National Drug Trade Conference*. Washington, DC: National Drug Trade Conference; 1989.

17. Cope JD. *The Story of the National Conference of Pharmaceutical Organizations*. Washington, DC: National Conference of Pharmaceutical Organizations; 1996.

18. Edwards WJ. Academy of General Practice of Pharmacy: a decade of service to the pharmacy practitioner. *J Am Pharm Assoc*. 1975;NS15: 322 4.

19. Florey KG. T*he Founding of the APhA Academy of Pharmaceutical Sciences: A History*. Washington, DC: American Pharmaceutical Association; 1979.

20. Cooper JF. *Twenty-Five Years—APhA Academy of Pharmacy Practice and Management Nuclear Pharmacy Section*. Washington, DC: American Pharmaceutical Association; 2000.

21. The pharmacist's role in product selection. *J Am Pharm Assoc*. 1971;NS11:181-99.

22. Palmieri A III. *Thirty Years of Scientific Excellence: APhA Academy of Pharmaceutical Research and Science*. Washington, DC: American Pharmaceutical Association; 1996.

23. 50th anniversary of APhA-ASP. *Pharmacy Student*. March/April 1999.

24. Pharmacy Technician Certification Board Web site. Available at: www.ptcb.org. Accessed January 24, 2002.

25. About AACP. American College of Clinical Pharmacy Web site. Available at: www.accp. com/about.html. Accessed January 24, 2002.

26. Comer B. Posey LM. *Twenty-Five Years of Caring: American Association of Consultant Pharmacists*. Alexandria, Va: American Association of Consultant Pharmacists; 1994.

27. Meade V. Specialization in pharmacy. *Am Pharm*. 1991; NS31 :24-9.

28. Cahill JA. History of the Academy of Managed Care Pharmacy. Poster presented at: American Pharmaceutical Association Annual Meeting; March 15-19, 2002; Philadelphia, Pa.

29. What is the background of PCMA and what is its origin? Pharmaceutical Care Management Association Web site. Available at: www.pcmanet.org/home. Accessed January 24, 2002.

30. Mount JK, Zellmer WA, Knowlton CH. Decade of pharmaceutical care. *Pharm Hist* 2001;43:66-92.

Name Index

A

Abbott, Walter 57
Abrams, Robert E. 51
Anderson, William C. 92
Arny, Henry Vincome 94
Avicenna 88
Ayer, James Cook 57

B

Beal, James H. 40, 93
Bectel, Maurice 73
Blauch, Lloyd E. 49
Borchardt, Ronald t. 32
Brodie, Don 14
Brown, Denny 92
Brown, Floyd W. 92
Burger, Warren 84

C

Carlin, Herb 73
Chen, K. K. 33, 73
Clark, Henry T., Jr. 51
Clinton, William Jefferson 16
Craigie, Andrew 55

D

Diehl, C. Lewis 88
Dohme, Charles Emile 92
Dohme, Louis 57
Dunn, Charles Wesley 63
Dunning, H. A. B. 65
Durham, Carl 11, 81

E

Eberhardt, Ernest G. 21
Ehrlich, Paul 25
Elliott, Edward C. 94

F

Feldman, Edward G. 32
Fischelis, Robert P. 50
Fischl, Louis J. 49
Francke, Don 14

G

Galen 88
Gibson, Melvin R. 14
Goyan, Jere E. 51, 73
Green, Melvin 94
Griffenhagen, George 22

H

Hallberg, Carl S. N. 40
Hardt, Robert 73
Hefley, Ed 92
Hepler, C. Douglas 16, 52, 106
Higby, Gregory 22
Higuchi, Takeru 29, 33
Hoffmann, Frederick 43
Holland, Madeline Oxford 50
Humphrey, Hubert 11, 13, 81
Hynson, Henry P. 92

J

Jones, David F. 92

K

Kefauver, Estes 106
Kelly, Evander F. 92,96
Kendall, Edward Calvin 27
Krantz, John C., Jr. 104
Kremers, Edward 40

L

Landsowne, J. Warren 72
Lederle, Ernst Joseph 62
Lemberger, Joseph 93
Liebenau, Jonathan 21
Liebig, Justus 88
Liggett, Louis K. 7
Lilly, Eli 57, 72, 73
Lilly, Josiah, Sr. 65
Lilly, Josiah K. 21
Lloyd, John Uri 57, 65
Lyman, Rufus 28
Lyons, Albert B. 21

M

MacCarney, John A. 72
Maisch, John M. 89
Mallinckrodt, Edward 65
Mario, Ernest 72
Marshall, Charles 55
Marshall, Christopher, Jr. 55
Miller, Jacob 73
Miller, William A. 52
Modell, J. Solon 95
Mrtek, Robert. 49

N

Nitardy, Fred 72
Nolan, Herman 13

O

Oldberg, Oscar 39, 40

P

Packard, Charles Herbert 94
Parrish, Edward 37, 87
Pelletier, Joseph Pierre 23
Pfeiffer, Gustavus 65

Power, Frederick B. 20, 39
Prescott, Albert B. 19, 38, 39
Procter, William, Jr. xi, 2, 22, 37

R

Reagan, Ronald 15
Remington, Joseph P. 40, 92
Rhudy, Marily 73
Richards, Richard Q. 49
Robins, E. Claiborne 72
Roosevelt, Theodore 62

S

Scheele, Carl 22,88
Smith, Daniel B. 13
Sonnedecker, Glenn 19, 20, 39
Squibb, E. R. 2
Stewart, Francis E. 40
Strand, Linda 16, 52

T

Teorell, Torsten 28
Tischler, Max 33
Tyler, Varro 33

U

Upjohn, William E. 57

W

Walgreen, Charles R. 7
Warner, William 57, 58
Weaver, Lawrence 73
Webster, George L. 49
Wellcome, Henry 65
Whelpley, Henry M. 43, 93, 94, 96
White, Eugene V. 13
Whitney, Harvey A. K. 95
Wiley, Harvey W. 62
Williams, Joseph 73
Wooten, Thomas 93
Wyeth, John 57